Fundamental aspects of

pain assessment and management

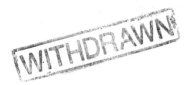

Other titles in the Fundamental Aspects of Nursing series include:

Adult Nursing Procedures edited by Penny Tremayne and Sam Parboteeah
Caring for the Person with Dementia by Kirsty Beart
Community Nursing edited by John Fowler
Complementary Therapies for Health Care Professionals by Nicky Genders
Gynaecology Nursing by Sandra Johnson
Legal, Ethical and Professional Issues in Nursing by Maggie Reeves and Jacquie Orford
Nursing Adults with Respiratory Disorders edited by Jane Scullion
Nursing the Acutely Ill Adult edited by Pauline Pratt
Men's Health by Morag Gray
Tissue Viability Nursing by Cheryl Dunford and Bridgit Günnewicht
Palliative Care Nursing by Robert Becker and Richard Gamlin
Women's Health by Morag Gray

Series Editor: John Fowler

Fundamental aspects of

pain assessment and management

edited by

Karina McGann

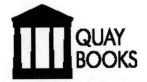

QUAY
BOOKS

Quay Books Division, MA Healthcare Ltd, St Jude's Church, Dulwich Road, London SE24 0PB

British Library Cataloguing-in-Publication Data
A catalogue record is available for this book

© MA Healthcare Limited 2007
ISBN 1 85642 292 5
ISBN 978 1 85642 292 5

Printed in the UK by Athenaeum Press Ltd., Gateshead, Tyne and Wear.

Contents

List of contributors   vii

Foreword   ix
Beverley Collett

Introduction   x
Karina McGann

1 The anatomy and physiology of pain   1
   Karina McGann
2 The pharmacological treatment of pain   11
   Karina McGann
3 The assessment of acute pain in adults   25
   Lorraine Buglass
4 The management of acute pain   37
   Angela Roberts
5 The assessment of chronic pain   51
   Kimberley Tordoff
6 The management of chronic non-malignant pain   63
   Lorraine Stevens
7 Pain in palliative care   77
   Gill Arnold, Jane Lee and Peter Stuart
8 The management of pain in children   95
   Sarah Roberts
9 Physiotherapy in the management of chronic pain   111
   Paul Watson
10 Psychological aspects of chronic pain treatment   125
   Kate Martin and Laura Ambrose
11 Complementary therapies and pain management   141
   Avril Holland

Index   159

Acknowledgements

The authors thank the following for their help and support in the writing of this book:

Sue Savage, medical secretary, for help with formatting; NAPP Pharmaceuticals for their sponsorship of the complementary therapy chapter; our spouses, partners, friends and work colleagues for their patience and support; and John Fowler for his continued guidance.

List of contributors

Laura Ambrose is Clinical Psychologist at University Hospitals of Leicester NHS Trust

Gill Arnold is Specialist Sister, Palliative Care at University Hospitals of Leicester NHS Trust

Lorraine Buglass is Nurse Specialist, Pain Management, University Hospitals of Leicester. NHS Trust

Avril Holland is Principal and Tutor at the Holland Academy of Complementary Therapies

Jane Lee is Specialist Sister, Palliative Care at University Hospitals of Leicester NHS Trust

Kate Martin is Assistant Psychologist at University Hospitals of Leicester NHS Trust

Karina McGann is Nurse Specialist, Pain Management at University Hospitals of Leicester NHS Trust

Angela Roberts is Nurse Specialist, Pain Management at University Hospitals of Leicester NHS Trust

Sarah Roberts is Children's Pain Specialist Nurse at the Children's Hospital, University Hospitals of Leicester NHS Trust

Lorraine Stevens is Nurse Specialist, Pain Management at University Hospitals of Leicester NHS Trust

Peter Stuart is Clinical Nurse Specialist, Palliative Care at University Hospitals of Leicester NHS Trust

Kimberley Tordoff is Nurse Specialist Pain Management at University Hospitals of Leicester NHS Trust

Paul Watson is Consultant Physiotherapist and Senior Lecturer, Department of Health Sciences at University of Leicester

Foreword

Beverley Collett

Pain is a universal human experience and its management is therefore fundamental to all health care professionals.

Nurses are the key professionals with whom the patient has closest contact. It is essential that nurses of all grades develop the necessary skills and competencies to assess and manage pain. This book will assist them on that path.

The book is primarily aimed at student and newly qualified nurses and gives a basic overview of all aspects of pain assessment and management. However, it can also be used by medical students, physiotherapists, psychologists and occupational therapists as it gives a basic overview of pain physiology and all aspects of pain management.

Innovative use of case studies and questions interplayed with informative text will help nurses think about the problem of pain within their specific clinical areas.

This book will help health care professionals in primary care, the community and secondary care to improve their management of pain. Pain is sometimes a symptom that resolves when disease is cured. However, it can persist in spite of treatment in those diseases for which there is no cure, or following trauma. Good management of pain is essential to improving the patient's quality of life. Nurses need to have knowledge of the advances being made in research in physiology, psychology and pharmacology, so that they are better able to assist in the management of their patient's pain and improve professional and patient education about this complex experience.

Beverley Collett is former President of the
British Pain Society of Great Britain and Ireland

Introduction

Karina McGann

Pain can have a devastating effect on a person's quality of life. A substantial proportion of the patients that health care professionals come into contact with suffer some sort of pain and this pain is not always related to the reason why the patient is consulting the health professional.

Inadequate assessment and knowledge are the most frequent reasons for poor pain management. Nurses play a vital role in both the assessment and management of pain. They can make a real difference in patients' lives by ensuring that their patients receive optimum levels of pain relief.

Providing information about a range of issues related to the many aspects of pain, this book is designed to introduce the reader to an overview of the different types of pain, the theory of pain and its assessment and subsequent management. The chapters are written by specialists who are actively involved in patient care within specific areas. The authors share their expert knowledge and hands on experience with the reader.

The book is intended to be read by student and newly qualified nurses and any other health care professionals who recognise a deficit in their knowledge. It can be read as a whole, giving sound knowledge on a broad spectrum of pain issues or it can be read by students who wish to update their knowledge in one specific area.

Chapter 1 introduces the reader to the basic science of pain. Anatomy and physiology are discussed relating theory to practice to enhance understanding. *Chapter 2* outlines the pharmacological treatments available across a broad spectrum including the unique role of the nurse in optimising analgesia.

Chapters 3 and 4 introduce the assessment and management of acute pain explaining the importance of treating acute pain quickly in order to prevent it from becoming chronic.

Chapters 5 and 6 introduce the assessment and management of chronic pain. *Chapter 7* gives an overview of the many aspects of pain in palliative care including assessment and management of the different types of malignant pain, including spiritual pain, and discusses ethical considerations.

Chapter 8 gives an overview of the assessment and treatment of pain in children, neonates and babies. Including pharmacological and non-pharmacological methods, it explains the importance of encompassing the needs of the whole child in order to improve pain relief.

Chapter 9 discusses the importance of physiotherapy in the long-term management of chronic pain.

Any patient in pain will have an emotional reaction to that pain, which can range from mild anxiety to severe distress, depression and negative thinking. *Chapter 10* identifies the psychological aspects of pain and why the use of psychological and behavioural techniques can assist with pain management.

Chapter 11 introduces the reader to the use of complementary therapies in the health care setting and discusses which therapies may be useful in the treatment of pain.

Each chapter links theory to practice. The use of case studies encourages readers to reflect on examples within their practice setting, thinking about how the patient's pain was managed and considering the issues involved. It is hoped that the time spent reflecting will help to influence and improve future pain management.

A summary of key points with implications for nursing practice are given at the end of each chapter.

This book is intended as an introduction to pain. It is hoped that it gives the reader an appetite to explore this challenging area of nursing in more depth and to use this knowledge to improve the management of patients in pain.

Karina McGann is Nurse Specialist, Pain Management at University
Hospitals of Leicester NHS Trust

CHAPTER I

The anatomy and physiology of pain

Karina McGann

What is pain?

Pain is an unpleasant sensory and emotional experience associated with actual or potential damage or described in terms of such damage (International Association for the Study of Pain, 1986). Inherent in this definition is the concept that pain always has a subjective component. It is both a physiological sensation and an emotional reaction to that sensation. It acknowledges the role that personal meaning and subjective experience play in the total pain experience.

There may be no tissue injury but the pain is no less 'real'. Pain is what the patient says it is (McCaffery, 1983). Pain is a common human fear. It is a protective mechanism for the body. Before we can begin to manage pain we need a basic understanding of functional anatomy and physiology. There are many routes and mechanisms of pain and these are often difficult to understand.

A good background knowledge can be used as a reference point when assessing, planning and implementing pain management. Greater understanding will lead to improvements in our ability to provide pain relief.

Acute pain

Acute pain is pain of sudden onset temporally related to injury and which resolves during the appropriate healing period. Acute pain often responds to treatment with analgesic medications and treatment of the precipitating cause.

Chronic pain

Chronic pain is often defined as pain that persists for more than three months after the usual healing process. Chronic non-malignant pain serves no useful biological purpose and is not necessarily a symptom of injury or disease. Chronic pain can be divided into two main types:

- nociceptive pain
- neuropathic pain.

Nociceptive pain

Nociception relates to the perception of a potentially tissue damaging (noxious) stimulus. It is the first step in the pain pathway. Nociceptive pain occurs after surgery or injury. The pain pathways are normal and the pain responds to standard analgesia.

Neuropathic pain

Neuropathic pain is associated with nerve damage. It may be due to an anatomical or functional abnormality of the pain pathway. Neuropathic pain is described by the patient as burning, shooting or a warm tingling. It responds poorly to standard analgesia and may benefit from the addition of adjuvants.

Pain receptors

Pain receptors are sometimes called nociceptors. Nociceptors are naked endings of Aδ and C fibres that carry impulses towards the central nervous system. Through them the body is able to detect the occurrence, location, intensity and duration of noxious stimuli and thereby signal the pain sensation. Pain receptors are located in the superficial layers of the skin and in internal tissues such as skeletal muscle, joint surfaces and periostium.

There are two types of pain receptor:

- The first type respond to mechanical deformation and distortion. These are described as high threshold mechanoreceptors (HTMs). They are present in the dermis of the skin.
- The second type respond to a variety of noxious inputs including mechanical injury, thermal irritation and chemical stimulation. These are polymodal nociceptors (PMNs).

Painful (tissue damaging) stimuli activate specific pain nociceptors in the tissues, which transduce noxious information into an electrical signal that is transmitted centrally. When stimulated, pain nociceptors are capable of exciting associated nerves.

Different nerve fibres are involved in the transmission of pain. Pain signals are transmitted from pain receptors in the skin along three types of nerve fibre.

Nerve fibres are classified according to size and whether or not they are surrounded by a coating of myelin. Myelination serves to insulate and speed up the conduction of impulses along the nerve.

Aδ fibres

Aδ fibres are rapidly conducting fibres that are thought to give rise to sensations of distinct sharp, well-defined and localised pain closely related to the time at which the external stimulus is received. This is often a warning signal and the receiver removes him or herself from the stimulation thus preventing further damage.

C fibres

The sharp stimulus is then followed by a duller more prolonged pain originating from C fibres. C fibres are thin slowly conducting fibres that are thought to give rise to the experience of diffuse, unpleasant and unbearable pain.

Aβ fibres

Aβ fibres carry other sensations, ie. information about vibration and position, from the periphery to the spinal cord.

Chemical neurotransmitters

Injury to tissues commonly results in inflammation which tends to be associated with pain. Chemical mediators are released when an inflammatory process occurs and C fibres are thought to be activated by some of these chemicals, which act as pain mediators. Enhancement or blocking of their action can potentially alter the way pain is mediated. These chemicals include noradrenaline, serotonin (5HT), substance P, bradykinin and prostaglandins.

STOP

Give an example of a treatment used within your area which may interrupt the release of one of the above chemicals.

Your answer is medication: NSAIDs are a common analgesic used to relieve musculoskeletal pain. They work by inhibiting the release of prostaglandin. Examples of NSAIDs include diclofenac, ibuprofen and meloxicam.

Endogenous opioid peptides

Endogenous opioids are morphine-like substances produced by the body in response to painful stimuli. The three main endogenous opioid peptides are enkephalin, endorphin and dynorphin. They are derived from biologically inactive peptide precursors and include approximately 20 peptides with opioid-like activity. The opioid peptides act as endogenous ligands for different types of opioid receptors (μ, δ and κ). Both opioid peptides and opioid receptors are distributed widely in the central nervous system within the sensory pathways that convey nociceptive information, ie. the sites associated with pain. The chemicals are thought to suppress conduction in the pain pathway.

The endogenous opioid peptides are thought to be activated by nociceptive stimuli and, as a consequence, an inhibitory modulation of sensory information occurs. Opioid drugs are manufactured to produce similar effects. Clinicians administer chemicals that mimic these substances in order to reduce pain.

STOP

Name one opioid drug used within your clinical area. What type of pain is it used for? Are there any other types of pain for which it could be used?

Transmission of pain through the spinal cord

Aδ and C fibres enter the spinal cord via the dorsal nerve roots and terminate on cells in the dorsal horn. The dorsal horn is a processing centre for incoming information. The information transmitted through Aδ and C fibres is significantly modified before transmission to the brain. The majority of nerve fibres enter the dorsal horn in the ventrolateral bundle of the dorsal root with 30% of the central processes of unmyelinated fibres entering through the ventral root. Both terminate in the dorsal horn of the cord.

The dorsal horn of the cord is divided into layers called laminae. The laminae are labelled I–V and have discrete functions related to pain processing. It is here that much of the modulation of pain transmission occurs.

Cells in lamina I, also called the marginal layer, are mainly excited by noxious, mechanical and thermal stimulation. Laminae II and III respond to the substantia geletanosa. Most of the Aδ and C fibres carrying the pain impulses synapse in the marginal zone and the substantia gelatinosa, although some Aδ fibres extend as far as lamina V. On entering the dorsal horn the nerve fibres synapse and then cross the middle of the cord to ascend to the brain.

Ascending pathways

The sensation of pain travels via the nerve fibres from the injury site to the spinal cord and then to the higher neurological centres, including the medulla, the midbrain, the thalamus and the limbic system

There are two main pathways which transmit from the spinal cord to the brain: the spinothalamic tract and the spinorecticular tract.

The spinothalamic tract

The majority of nerve fibres carrying pain impulses ascend in the spinothalamic tract. As its name suggests the spinothalamic tract connects the spinal nerves with the thalamus mostly carrying information about the position and quality of pain. The thalamus sits below the cerebral hemisphere and is the key area for the processing of somatosensory information. Some fibres in the medial thalamus project to the periaqueductal grey matter, the reticular formation and the hypothalamus; these fibres are thought to be involved in the autonomic and motivational aspects of pain.

The spinorecticular tract

The spinorecticular tract has a much wider distribution and is less easily localised. It projects to the thalamus, hypothalamus and the limbic system and is responsible for a wide spectrum of pain sensations from light pressure to severe pain. It probably accounts for the emotional aspects of chronic pain.

The perception of pain

All neurones transmitting pain eventually synapse in the thalamus. Nerve pathways run from the thalamus to the sensory cortex. Here the information is analysed further and this explains how knowledge and memory of previous pain experience and cultural influences have an effect on the perception of pain. This helps to explain why two patients having the same operation report different levels of pain post-operatively.

Axons in the spinothalamic tract also synapse with the medulla, hypothalamus and the limbic system before reaching the thalamus. This pathway is important in determining an individual's emotional reaction to pain. The medulla probably helps to initiate the response of the autonomic nervous system to painful stimuli, eg. the initiation of nervous impulses resulting in muscular contraction so that movement occurs away from the source of pain.

Descending modulation

All nociceptive ascending transmission is capable of being modified by descending neural control from the brain. As well as pain pathways that ascend from the peripheries via the spinal cord to the brain there are other nerve fibres that descend from the brain. When activated these result in a reduction in perceived pain.

The cerebral aqueduct is a narrow canal in the midbrain connecting the thalamus to the cerebellum. The grey matter surrounding the aqueduct, the periaqueductal grey (PAG) receives input from the thalamus, the hypothalamus,

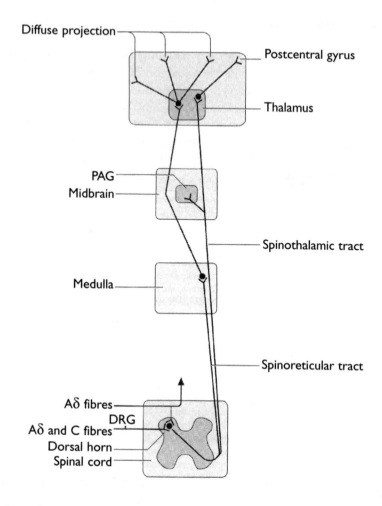

Figure 1.1: Ascending and descending pain pathways. PAG: periaqueductal grey; DRG dorsal root ganglion.

the cortex and the collaterals from the spinothalamic tract and so is an important centre for descending control of pain. This area can activate descending pathways which can inhibit the nociceptive stimulus. This probably happens in the early synapses in the dorsal horn. Nerves within the pathways use neurotransmitters, mainly serotonin and noradrenaline, the action of which can be modified by drugs. See *Figure 1.1* for a diagrammatic representation of ascending and descending pathways.

STOP

Give an example of a drug that may be prescribed for pain which may enhance or inhibit the action of serotonin.

Amitriptyline, a common antidepressant drug, is known to inhibit the reuptake of serotonin and is commonly prescribed for the treatment of neuropathic pain. You can read more about this in Chapters 2 and 4 on pharmacology and chronic pain management.

The gate theory of pain

Postulated by Melzack and Wall (1965), in its simplest form the gate theory of pain suggests that the dorsal horn acts as a gate for the control of painful sensations into the ascending neurones. If the gate can be closed the painful sensations can be modified. The basic premises are that activity in large (non-nociceptive) fibres can inhibit the perception of that activity in small (nociceptive) fibres, and that descending activity from the brain can also inhibit that perception. For example, rubbing a painful area stimulates Aβ fibres which then inhibit the spinal synapses of A and C fibres. Consequently, less input is delivered to the ascending pathways and less pain is perceived. The gate is closed.

STOP

Consider any treatments that are currently used or could be used within your clinical area which may improve pain relief by closing the pain gate.

Anything that helps the patient to feel better will close the pain gate. Your answer may have included reassurance, medication, transcutaneous electrical nerve stimulation, relaxation therapy and complementary therapies.

How the nervous system alters in response to injury

When asked about their pain patients sometimes report pain levels higher than would normally be expected and that it appears more widespread than the damage causing it. To the health care professional the injury has healed and an assumption is made that the pain is better. However, this is often not the case.

This may be due to prolonged stimulation of the dorsal horn cells within the spinal cord and the increase in their response exacerbates the patient's perception of pain. When an injury is inflicted pain is first evoked by the stimulation of the nociceptors and the release of algesic substances in a localised area. Inflammation sensitises the nociceptors making them far more sensitive to stimulation, this is known as hyperalgesia. Hyperalgesia felt at the site of stimulation is known as primary hyperalgesia and it is related to sensitisation of the neurones innervating that area. To the patient there is a perception that a normally painful stimulus is more painful than usual. As healing begins nerve endings of the polymodal C fibres show increased response to stimuli. The fibres become more easily stimulated and what would have previously been perceived as an innocuous stimulus to Aβ fibres becomes a painful condition known as secondary hyperalgesia. Such changes result in fewer stimuli proving painful and lasting longer with pain felt by the patient not at the site of their original injury but in a surrounding area of normal healthy tissue. The dorsal horn cells can continue firing long after the initial stimulus has stopped and long after the normal healing period.

The physiological consequence of these changes is hyperexcitability of the dorsal horn neurone. This is often referred to as wind up. Wind up will occur following all injuries but may be particularly important following long-term nociceptor activity (eg. in degenerative back pain) or damage to nerves themselves which leads to abnormal messages being transmitted (Dalgleish, 2000). Prolonged wind up may result in an acute pain becoming chronic. It is believed that N-methyl-D-aspartate acid (NMDA) receptors could be responsible for the wind up phenomenon. Antagonists of NMDA receptors such as ketamine may have a role in the treatment of pain.

Conclusion

Pain reaches consciousness following a series of complex routes to and from the brain. The sensation of pain can be blocked or enhanced by chemical neurotransmitters or interruption of the ascending signal by closure of the pain gate. Nurses have a unique role to play in the interruption of the ascending pathway by initiating treatments that block or enhance neurotransmitters and by closing the pain gate.

Implications for nursing practice

- Believe patients when they say they are in pain.
- Early initiation of treatment may interrupt the pain pathway and prevent acute pain from becoming chronic.

Key points

- Pain is a sensory and emotional experience.
- Pain reaches consciousness due to a series of ascending and descending mechanisms.
- Chemical pain mediators are thought to be released during the inflammatory process.
- The gate theory of pain helps to explain descending mechanisms.
- Pain is what the patient says it is even in the absence of tissue damage.
- Greater understanding of the above will lead to improvements in pain relief.

References

Dalgleish D (2000) Anatomy and physiology of pain. In Munafo M, Trim J (Eds.) *Chronic Pain. A handbook for Nurses*. Butterworth Heinemann: Oxford.

International Association for the Study of Pain (1986) *Classification of Chronic Pain. Descriptions of Chronic Pain*. International Association for the Study of Pain: Seattle, WA.

McCaffery M (1983) *Nursing Management of the Patient in Pain*. JB Lippincott Co: Philadelphia.

Melzack R, Wall PD (1965) Pain mechanisms: A new theory. *Science* **150**(699): 971–9.

Stannard C, Booth S (2004) *Pain* (2nd edn) Elsevier Churchill Livingstone: Oxford.

CHAPTER 2

The pharmacological treatment of pain

Karina McGann

The pharmacological treatment of pain should be considered as one component of a treatment plan. A full and detailed assessment of the quality of the pain as well as its intensity should be carried out prior to prescribing.

Routes of delivery

Drugs can be delivered by many routes

- oral
- sublingual
- rectal
- subcutaneous
- intramuscular
- intravenous
- transdermal
- buccal
- intra-articular.

The route of administration influences a drug's absorption and distribution. Each route has advantages and disadvantages.

Oral
The oral route is the most convenient and easiest way to take analgesics. Drugs are absorbed from the gastrointestinal tract and are generally available in tablet, capsule and liquid forms.

Sublingual
The drug is placed under the tongue and most drugs administered in this way are rapidly disintegrating tablets or soft gelatine capsules. A high concentration of the drug is achieved in the sublingual region before it is absorbed by the mucosa. Absorption can be unpredictable.

Rectal
Drugs can be given rectally as a suppository. Onset is slow and there is variable absorption.

Subcutaneous
Subcutaneous drugs are injected into fatty tissue beneath the skin. Drug absorption and action depend on the specific drug and its properties. Subcutaneous medication can be given through single injection or via a patient analgesia pump. Absorption is slower than via the intramuscular route.

Intramuscular
Intramuscular injections deliver medication deep into muscle tissue. This route is often used when the subcutaneous, oral or intravenous routes are unavailable. Absorption is dependent on the drug and factors such as exercise and rubbing the site of administration. Pain and irritation at the injection site are common.

Intravenous
Drugs given via a vein have a rapid onset as the drug enters the blood stream directly. The drug is absorbed rapidly but has a short duration of action.

Transdermal
In the transdermal route creams, gels, ointments or patches are applied to the skin and the drug is absorbed through the skin thereby by-passing the liver. This route is useful for slow-release preparations. Absorption can be variable.

Buccal
In buccal administration a tablet is inserted between the cheek and the mouth. Because the buccal mucosa is less permeable than the sublingual area, absorption is slower and drug availability is decreased.

Intra-articular
Intra-articular administration delivers the drug directly to the synovial joint cavity. It can achieve pain relief, reduce inflammation and produce numbness.

Patient controlled analgesia

In selected patients patient controlled analgesia (PCA) devices may be used to deliver intravenous, subcutaneous or intrathecal medication, primarily opioids. PCA can promote independence and reduce the need for repeated titration of medication by health care professionals. Appropriate patient selection is important and patients who can tolerate oral medication may not require PCA.

Pharmacokinetics

As has been detailed, drugs may be given to patients in various ways; they may be injected, absorbed from the gastrointestinal tract after oral or rectal administration, applied locally or inhaled.

The term bioavailabilty is used to denote the proportion of the administered dose of the drug that reaches the circulation. If a drug is given intravenously then the bioavailabilty is 100%; if it is swallowed then only a proportion may reach the circulation.

First-pass metabolism

Drugs absorbed from the gastrointestinal tract enter the portal venous blood supply and pass through the liver before entering the systemic circulation. This is know as first-pass hepatic metabolism and explains the reason for large differences in effect between oral and intravenous drugs that undergo extensive hepatic extraction and metabolism. The extent of first-pass metabolism of any drug may vary greatly between individuals, and this may account for the large range of doses of the same drug needed by different patients.

Protein binding

A term used frequently in pharmacology is protein binding. When a drug is taken a variable amount is bound to plasma proteins. Protein binding has an important effect on the distribution of drugs because only the free or unbound fraction is readily available to cross the cell membrane and so have a pharmacological action.

The volume distribution of a drug is related to protein binding. Clearance of a drug is also influenced by protein binding because it is the unbound fraction in the plasma that has ready access to first-pass metabolism and undergoes glomerular filtration.

The drug protein complex is maintained by a weak bond and can dissociate when the plasma concentration of a drug declines as a result of hepatic or renal clearance of the unbound drug.

Alterations in protein binding are important for drugs that are highly protein bound. If a drug is 75% protein bound and this decreases to 73%, the plasma concentration of this unbound drug will double with potential associated increases in pharmacological effects. A decrease in protein binding results in an increase in the free fraction of a drug. The extent of protein binding parallels lipid solubility of the drug. In addition to this the fraction of total drug that is protein bound in the plasma is determined by the drug's plasma concentration and the number of available binding sites. Low plasma concentrations of drugs are likely to be more highly protein bound than are higher plasma concentrations of the same drug.

Renal failure may decrease the fraction of the drug bound to protein even in the absence of a change of plasma concentration. This may be due to a metabolic factor excreted by the kidney displacing the drug, or an alteration in protein structure. Some proteins such as albumin tend to be present in lower levels in the elderly.

The pharmacokinetics and pharmacodynamics of drugs can provide interesting reading. Further information can be obtained from pharmacological textbooks for those students who wish to develop their knowledge.

General prescribing principles

The WHO ladder

The World Health Organization (WHO) developed a series of guidelines to address deficiencies in the treatment of cancer pain (World Health Organization, 1986). The central component of these guidelines is the analgesic three-step ladder (*Figure 2.1*). The concept behind the analgesic ladder is broad spectrum analgesia, eg. drugs from each of the classes of analgesia are used appropriately, either singly or in combination to maximise there impact. If treatment is ineffective the patient is moved up a step.

The guidelines suggest that, if pain occurs, there should be prompt administration of a drug in the following order until the patient is free of pain and not suffering with intolerable side-effects:

- non-opioid
- mild opioid
- strong opioid.

The analgesic ladder does not have an upper limit since there is no maximum dose for strong opioids. If pain remains a problem despite high doses of strong opioid or the side-effects are severe, the cause of pain should be reassessed and/or further specialist advice should be obtained. Patients who do not respond despite escalating doses may not have an opioid-responsive pain. Different types of pain require different types of therapy, and additional drugs called adjuvants can be used.

The WHO advises that, for effective pain relief, analgesia is best given

- by the clock
- by mouth
- the right drug
- in the right dose at the right time.

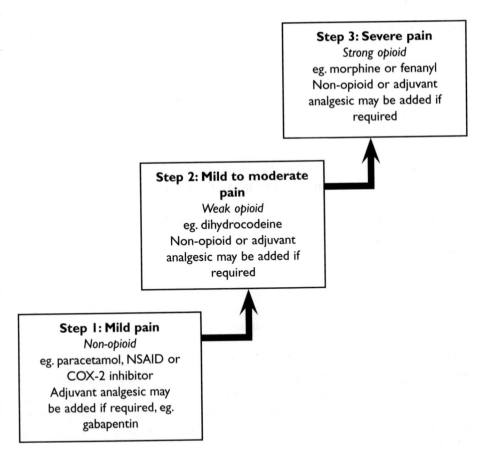

Figure 2.1: The WHO analgesic ladder. NSAID, non-steroidal anti-inflammatory drug; COX-2, cyclo-oxygenase 2.

The guidelines suggested by the WHO should be considered good practice by all nurses involved in the administration of medicines. The ladder is now used more widely than just for cancer pain; it acts as a cornerstone for many pain management guidelines.

STOP

Consider the differences you might consider when using the ladder in acute pain and chronic pain.

Your answer should discuss that for acute pain treatment may start with a strong opioid and work down the ladder as the pain improves and for chronic pain treatment may start with a weak/moderate opioid and work up the ladder if the pain does not respond.

Types of analgesia

Non-opioid analgesics

Non-opioid analgesics include paracetamol, aspirin and non-steroidal anti-inflammatory drugs (NSAIDs).

Paracetamol

Paracetamol is a widely used minor analgesic. Its mode of action is not fully understood but it is mediated by action on the central nervous system. It does not cause indigestion or gastric bleeding. Side-effects are uncommon at normal dosage but overdose can cause serious liver damage.

Aspirin

Aspirin is effective in pain of low intensity and has the advantage of having anti-inflammatory properties. Its side-effects include effects on the 8th cranial nerve such as tinnitus, deafness, dizziness and vomiting, gastric irritation, and bronchospasm in hypersensitive patients.

NSAIDs

NSAIDs are a large group of drugs and are the most commonly purchased over-the-counter medication. NSAIDs are recognised as important in the treatment of both acute and chronic pain. They are indicated for pain from inflammation and may also be used in non-inflammatory conditions (American Pain Society, 2003).

NSAIDs are believed to act by suppressing the formation within the peripheral tissues of prostaglandins which occur naturally and are released by cell damage. One of the actions of prostaglandins is concerned with the production of painful stimuli and they are also responsible for many of the features of inflammation.

Two enzymes, cyclo-oxygenase 1 (COX-1) and cyclo-oxygenase 2 (COX-2) are concerned with the formation of prostaglandins. Prostaglandins provided by COX-2 are responsible for pain and inflammation whereas those from COX-1 have a protective effect on the stomach lining. NSAIDs block both COX-1 and COX-2 and may relieve pain but also increase the risk of stomach ulcers.

NSAIDs that inhibit only COX-2 have fewer gastro-intestinal side-effects but may have other side-effects. One group has recently been withdrawn due to cardiac toxicity. NSAIDs account for more reports of toxicity than any other type of agent (Hawkey, 2002). They are responsible for multiple side-effects. Careful patient selection and a full medical assessment is essential.

The National Institute for Health and Clinical Excellence (NICE) has clear guidelines on which NSAID is the most appropriate to prescribe for which condition (for further reading visit the NICE website).

Side-effects of NSAIDs include gastric bleeding and perforation due to inhibition of the gastric protective action of prostaglandins. Care should be taken in elderly patients and patients who a report a previous history of peptic ulceration.

Renal toxicity is another side-effect of NSAIDs. NSAIDs rarely cause damage to the kidneys in normal patients. However, in patients with heart failure, cirrhosis of the liver, renal disease or who are taking diuretics they can occasionally precipitate renal failure. This is believed to be due to an alteration of blood flow through the kidneys which follows inhibition of prostaglandin production. Renal function should be monitored closely in this group of patients.

Haematological side-effects can also occur. Most NSAIDs inhibit platelet aggregation. Bleeding time will be prolonged requiring consideration in some patients especially in the pre-operative period.

NSAIDs are contra-indicated in patients with a hypersensitivity to aspirin and in patients with a history of peptic ulceration. They should be used with caution in elderly people, pregnant women, breastfeeding mothers, patients with coagulation problems and those with a history of hepatic or renal problems, cardiac insufficiency, or asthma.

COX-1 NSAIDs include ibuprofen, voltarol, and indomethacin. COX-2 NSAIDs include celebrex, meloxicam and ketorolac.

STOP

A 40-year-old man is admitted to an acute medical ward suffering with acute low back pain. The pain came on suddenly while he was lifting at work. X-ray and neurological examination indicate no disc prolapse or serious pathology.
He is to be prescribed a non-opioid analgesic and an NSAID.
What would you need to know before deciding which NSAID to prescribe?

You would need to know whether he had previously suffered with any cardiac, renal or gastro-intestinal problems and whether he is asthmatic or has any known allergies to medication.

Opioid analgesics

Types of opioid have not changed substantially over recent years. Morphine remains the most common drug of choice. Indications for use of opioids include post-operative pain, acute pain of moderate to severe intensity, cancer pain and chronic non-malignant pain.

The use of opioid therapy in chronic non-malignant pain is controversial and fear of addiction often prevents the prescribing of opioids in this group of patients. The British Pain Society has established a series of guidelines for the use of opiates in non-cancer pain which can be accessed on their website (www. britishpainsociety.org).

The mode of action of opioids mimics the action of three endogenous pain-killing peptides (endorphins, dynorphins and enkephalins). They bind to three receptors (μ, κ and δ) and block the release of neurotransmitters such as substance P.

Opioids are classified as full agonists and partial or mixed agonists. Full agonists usually bind to μ receptors and include codeine, morphine, hydromorphine, methadone and fentanyl. Partial or mixed agonists bind to more than one receptor and include buprenorphine, tramadol and nalbuphine.

Naloxone is a pure antagonist, it has no stimulating actions and no analgesic action. It reverses the effect of natural and synthetic opioids and is used in the treatment of opioid overdose.

The advantages of using opioids include the fact that, unlike non-opioid analgesics, full opioid agonists have no ceiling effect. Opioid doses can be titrated upwards until satisfactory pain control is achieved or side-effects become intolerable.

Opioids are contraindicated in acute respiratory depression, acute alcoholism, previous history of opiate abuse or sensitivity, paralytic illeus, acute abdomen and raised intracranial pressure. They should be used with caution in patients with asthma or decreased respiratory reserve and convulsive disorders, and in elderly patients and those with debilitated hepatic impairment.

Side-effects of opioids include respiratory depression, sedation, constipation, dry mouth, bradycardia, dysphoria and hallucinations. Some side-effects can be minimised with prophylactic therapy.

Opioids come in several dosage forms including oral, rectal and transdermal meeting the needs of many groups of patients. Constant pain requires round-the-clock rather than 'as required' medication. Doses should be adjusted/titrated until relief occurs with tolerable side-effects.

Breakthrough analgesia should be given to assist titration and prior to painful procedures. A short-acting opioid 10–15% of the total daily dose and not required more than four times a day should be given. Increments in the daily dose reflect breakthrough and reduce the need.

Adjuvant drugs include some antidepressants, anticonvulsants, systemically administered local anaesthetics, corticosteriods and N-methyl-D-aspartate acid (NMDA) antagonists. Used at any of the three steps of the analgesic ladder they can enhance the effects of opioids or provide analgesia for specific types of pain. Many of the adjuvant drugs are used beyond licence (or marketing authorisation) (Bennett and Simpson, 2002).

Tricyclic antidepressant drugs

Many of the neurotransmitters involved in nociception are affected by tryciclic antidepressants (TCAs) particularly the reuptake of serotonin and noradrenaline. TCAs do not produce pain relief by reversing co-existing depression since pain relief occurs at much lower doses than those required to treat depression. In some patients the effects of the drugs on sleep or lightened mood improves the ability to cope with the pain.

Amitriptyline is the most commonly prescribed drug in this group. There is more research with amitriptyline than any other antidepressant drug. Other drugs include venlafaxine, imipramine and duloxetine.

Contra-indications to the use of TCAs include acute myocardial infarction, coronary insufficiency, heart block, lactation, pregnancy, mania and severe liver disease.

Abrupt withdrawal should be avoided and TCAs should be used with caution in patients with cardiovascular disease, diabetes, epilepsy, glaucoma, hepatic impairment, urinary retention or thyroid disease and in elderly patients.

Side-effects include drowsiness, dry mouth, arrhythmias and heart block, constipation, urine retention, sweating, convulsions, hepatic reactions and blurred vision. Side-effects often limit the dose patients receive. In general starting doses should be low and the dose should be titrated up slowly until pain is controlled. Patients need to have a careful explanation that side-effects will occur before pain relief and that they may last 7–10 days.

Anticonvulsants

A number of anticonvulsants can be used in the treatment of pain. Their mode of action is different from antidepressants. They probably help pain control through different mechanisms, which are thought to suppress paroxysmal discharges and other abnormal neural transmission by stabilising neural membranes and reducing neuronal excitability.

The use of anticonvulsants is contra-indicated in patients with atrioventricular conduction abnormalities, a history of bone marrow depression, women who are lactating and in patients with myasthenia gravis or porphyria.

Anticonvulsants should be used with caution in patients with glaucoma, cardiac disease or a history of psychotic illness, patients undergoing haemodialysis, or elderly patients.

Side-effects of anticonvulsants include nausea, rashes, ataxia, dizziness, headaches, confusion, fatigue and tremor.

Common anticonvulsants include gabapentin, carbamazapine, pregabalin and phenytoin.

Anti-arrhythmics

Anti-arrhythmics have been found to be useful in the treatment of neuropathic pain. They work by suppressing aberrant electrical activity in central neurones and damaged peripheral axons by blocking sodium channels.

They are contra-indicated in patients with sino-atrial disorders, all grades of atrioventricular block and myocardial depression. They should be used with caution in patients with congestive cardiac failure or hepatic impairment and in elderly patients.

Side-effects of anti-arrhythmics include ataxia, atrial fibrillation, blood disorders, bradycardia, conduction defects, confusion, constipation, convulsions, dizziness and drowsiness.

Although not licensed for use in pain both lignocaine and mexiletine have been used based on clinical experience and experimental evidence (Mimms, 2006).

Corticosteroids

Corticosteroids reduce oedema and the production of inflammatory mediators of pain by the direct inhibition of spontaneous activity in excitory damaged nerves.

Contra-indications include the presence of systemic infections. They should be used with caution in patients with adrenal suppression, infection, hypertension, recent myocardial infarction, liver failure, liver impairment, diabetes mellitus, osteoporosis, glaucoma, epilepsy, peptic ulceration, hypothyroidism, history of severe myopathy and pregnancy, and in children and adolescents.

Side-effects include aseptic necrosis of the femoral and humoral head, central nervous system disturbances, cushingoid changes, depression, euphoria, gastro-intestinal effects, osteoporosis and glaucoma.

Common corticosteroids include dexamethasone, hydrocortisone, methylprednisolone, prednisolone and betamethasone.

Anti-spasmodic/muscle relaxant drugs

This group of drugs act peripherally on the central nervous system. They are contra-indicated in patients with peptic ulceration and should be used with caution in patients with renal impairment, psychiatric illness, Parkinson's disease, cerebrovascular disease or epilepsy and in elderly patients.

Side-effects include sedation, drowsiness, muscular hypotonia, nausea, urinary disturbances, ataxia, hypotension, respiratory depression and dry mouth.

Commonly used anti-spasmodic/muscle relaxant drugs include baclofen, buscopan and diazepam.

Topical preparations

Capsaicin is used in the treatment of pain. It works by depleting local sensory nerve terminals of substance P. It produces desensitisation after initial excitation.

Contact with the eyes and inflamed or broken skin should be avoided. Capsaicin should never be used under tight bandages and patients should avoid taking a hot shower or a bath just before or after application.

Side-effects may include a transient burning sensation.

Nerve blocks

Injections of local anaesthetic, steroids, or neurolytic agents (chemical agents) can be administered into nerves, nerve plexuses or local trigger points.

These injections act by interrupting the nociceptive input at its source or by blocking nociceptive impulses in peripheral nerve fibres. They may interrupt the afferent and efferent limbs of abnormal reflex mechanisms and block the unmyelinated C and B fibres and small Aδ fibres. Blocking of sodium channels prevents action potentials and so decreases sensation arising in the affected area.

Side-effects include shivering, confusion, twitching, tremor, numbness and motor block.

Examples of drugs used for nerve block include lignocaine, bupivacaine, prilocaine and depo-medrone.

Spinal opioids

Spinal opioids can be administed via the epidural or intrathecal route.

- Epidural administration: The drug is administered into the epidural space. The drug can be given as a bolus dose or via an indwelling catheter to provide relief to irritated nerves. Drugs that can be given via this route include opioids, local anaesthetics, narcotics and steroids. Drawbacks include infection, bleeding and site tenderness.
- Intrathecal administration: In the intrathecal route the drug is administered into the subarachnoid space of the spinal canal. It is used to administer drugs that do not cross the blood-brain barrier. Morphine, baclofen, clonidine and some anaesthetics are given to achieve regional anaesthesia, spinal analgesia or epidural block in chronic pain and cancer pain.

The intrathecal and epidural routes are effective for providing analgesia. Opioids can be infused alone or in combination with other agents such as local anaesthetics or an α2 agonist such as clonidine. Fentanyl and morphine are the most commonly used. Agents can be administered as a single bolus or as a continuous infusion.

Spinal opioids are used peri-operatively and post-operatively and can also be used for cancer pain and chronic pain when a sufficient trial of systemic opioids has failed to control pain or when intolerable side-effects have occurred.

Risks of this route include nausea, itching and urinary retention. Reported serious adverse effects include infection, respiratory depression, and epidural haematoma.

The role of the nurse in pharmacology

Pharmacology plays a major role in the treatment of pain. Patients generally turn to the nurse for relief of their pain and nurses are in a prime position to ensure that patients receive analgesia quickly and repeatedly.

Individual assessment ensures that patients receive analgesia based on their needs and nurses are in the best position to provide this because they spend more time with the patient than any other health care professional. Liaison with the medical practitioner or nurse prescriber ensures that the most appropriate drugs are prescribed and choosing which drug to administer when more than one has been prescribed is the unique role of the nurse. The choice of drug should be based on using the lowest effective dose for maximum effect and minimum side-effects.

Personal development helps nurses to keep their knowledge updated and understand how drugs work and how combinations of drugs can provide a more balanced analgesia. Once administered it is the responsibility of the nurse to undertake regular re-evaluation and ensure that appropriate changes to drug regimens are made quickly and side-effects are eased.

Educating patients about the benefits of good pain control will help to achieve concordance. Patients need to understand the purpose of therapy in order to comply with the treatment. Advice about the dose and potential side-effects is essential as well as correction of misconceptions about fear of addiction.

The growth of nurse prescribing is an asset to the role of the nurse and will only benefit the administration of medicines. Prescribing decisions being made at the time of the problem and not when a doctor is available to alter the prescription will not only enhance patient care but will also result in patients receiving analgesia and subsequent pain relief in a much more timely and acceptable manner.

Implications for nursing practice

- Nurses have a unique role to play in the administration of medicines.
- Analgesia should be given regularly and not as required.
- Full explanation of the drugs and possible side-effects should be given to the patient.

Key points

- The initiation of medication should be considered as one component of a multidisciplinary treatment plan.
- All patients will need a full assessment before prescribing or administration decisions are made.
- The oral route is the easiest and most convenient and should be used whenever possible.
- Following treatment patients should be re-evaluated regularly and prompt changes made if treatment is ineffective or side-effects become intolerable.
- If patients are not obtaining pain relief despite escalating doses then different types of drugs may need to be considered.

References

American Pain Society (2003) *Principles of Analgesic Use in the Treatment of Acute Pain and Cancer Pain* (5th edn.) American Pain Society: Glenview, Il.

Bennett M, Simpson K (2002) The use of drugs beyond licence in palliative care and pain management. *Palliative Med* **16**(5): 367–8.

Hawkey CJ (2002) Cyclo-oxygenase inhibition; between the devil and the deep blue sea. *Gut* **50**(Suppl 3): iii25–30.

Mims (2006) *Mims Handbook of Pain Management* (4th edn) Medical Imprint on behalf of NAPP Pharmaceuticals: Cambridge.

World Health Organization (1986) *Cancer Pain Relief.* World Health Organization: Geneva.

Further reading

McCaffery M (1983) *Nursing Management of the Patient in Pain.* JB Lippincott Co: Philadelphia.

McCarberg B, Passik SD (2005) *Expert Guide To Pain Management.* American College of Physicians: Philadelphia.

Trounce J (2000) *Clinical Pharmacology for Nurses* (16th edn) Churchill Livingstone: Edinburgh.

Useful websites

www.britishpainsociety.org

www.iasp-pain.org

www.nice.org.uk

CHAPTER 3

The assessment of acute pain in adults

Lorraine Buglass

Introduction

Pain is a subjective, complex and multifaceted experience, and in order to manage it appropriately accurate assessment is essential. This chapter focuses on the principles of acute pain assessment.

What is acute pain?

Acute pain refers to pain that is of sudden onset and, usually, of limited duration. Examples of acute pain include pain from surgery, trauma, burns, myocardial infarction, renal colic and labour pain.

It has been said that pain is whatever the experiencing person says it is and it exists whenever the experiencing person says it does. This is because the pain experience is always subjective, and depends on physiological and psychological factors. Furthermore, there is no measure for detecting the amount of pain an individual experiences and thus the most accurate measurement must be taken from the individual's self-report.

Why assess?

The assessment of acute pain is fundamental to the diagnosis, management and treatment of any person with an acute condition. Failure to undertake assessment of the individual's pain experience may lead to misdiagnosis and inappropriate or inadequate treatment of pain. Without assessment one cannot determine whether treatment is necessary, effective or whether it should be discontinued. In addition, uncontrolled acute pain has been attributed to a number of adverse outcomes.

Effects of untreated acute severe pain

Unrelieved acute pain increases the risk of complications that can be life-threatening, especially in older people with pre-existing medical conditions.

Respiratory system

Severe chest or abdominal pain can result in splinting of the abdominal and chest wall muscles that can lead to decreased lung volumes and decreased ability to cough. This in turn may result in sputum retention, infection and hypoxaemia (Hamill, 1994).

Cardiovascular system

Severe pain increases sympathetic nervous system activity that results in tachycardia, hypertension, and increased myocardial oxygen consumption which may lead to myocardial ischaemia. Increased peripheral vascular resistance and altered regional blood flow towards the brain and heart may lead to poor wound healing and increased muscle spasm (Cousins and Power, 1999).

Neuroendocrine system

Severe pain is believed to cause an increase in the release of catecholamines, cortisol, glucagon, vasopressin, growth hormone, aldosterone and insulin. This is referred to as the 'stress response' and can lead to hyperglycaemia and increased fibrinogen and platelet activation, thus increasing blood coagulability which raises the risk of deep vein thrombosis (DVT) and pulmonary embolism (PE) (Cousins and Power, 1999). Furthermore, increased protein breakdown and negative nitrogen balance result in impaired immune function and wound healing, and sodium and fluid retention.

Gastro-intestinal and genito-urinary system

Severe pain has been associated with an increased incidence of nausea and vomiting, delays in gastric emptying, reduced gut motility and urinary retention (Hamill, 1994).

Musculoskeletal system

Pain not only causes muscle spasms and splinting, but also results in decreased mobility. This in turn increases the risk of DVT and PE.

Psychology

Untreated pain can result in increased anxiety, fear, agitation, withdrawal, insomnia and resentment or distrust of health care workers.

Central nervous system

Untreated acute severe pain can lead to central sensitisation (wind up) of the dorsal horn within the spinal cord (see *Chapter 1*). This in turn can lead to increased sensitisation to painful stimuli and has been linked to chronic pain.

Assessment

The British Pain Society advocates assessment of pain as the fifth vital sign, along with blood pressure, pulse, temperature and respiratory rate.

The goal of acute pain management is to prevent or intervene aggressively to keep pain to a minimum and to avoid the deleterious effects of uncontrolled pain. In order to do this we must assess accurately and to facilitate this we must understand when, what and how to assess.

A number of studies have demonstrated that health care workers do not rate pain intensity as accurately as patients themselves (Seers, 1987; Watt-Watson, 1987; Briggs and Dean, 1998). Health care workers need to be aware that they may inadvertently introduce bias when assisting patients to use a pain assessment tool and therefore need to be mindful of their role in educating patients about their use and ensure that it is the patient's perspective that is recorded (Bird, 2003).

Factors affecting the assessment of pain

There are multiple factors that may influence the assessment of acute pain, these include: patient, health care worker and environmental factors.

Patient factors that may influence assessment include:

- fear and anxiety
- previous experience
- personality
- culture
- age
- knowledge
- sleep disruption
- illness
- the environment and the response of those around the patient.

Health care worker factors include:

- personal beliefs and biases
- personal experience
- knowledge of pain physiology, pain assessment tools, and analgesia.

Patients and in particular older patients may be reluctant to report pain to the health care worker, and therefore sensitive questioning is required. Effective communication in a trusting nurse–patient relationship is essential to help people express their pain. Patients need to feel that an expression of pain will be listened to, accepted and acted upon (Closs, 1994).

When should pain be assessed?

Pain should be assessed on admission to hospital or prior to admission, ie. at a pre-assessment clinic. This enables a baseline to be established and information to be gained about how the individual usually copes with pain including pharmacological and non-pharmacological coping strategies. Previous experiences and expectations may be useful in developing the patient's pain management care plan. It also provides an opportunity to clear up any misconceptions and to influence patients' expectations of how pain can be managed. The suitability of particular pain assessment tools and management techniques can be established according to cognitive function, age, and functional ability.

After the initial baseline assessment, pain should be assessed according to patients' needs, but at least as frequently as their vital signs. In order to assess efficacy of any treatment strategy, pain must be reassessed within an appropriate time frame of analgesia administration. It may be appropriate to wait 30–45 minutes to assess the effects of weak opiates or paracetamol in a patient with mild to moderate pain, however, this time-frame would be inappropriate if a patient was in the emergency department with severe pain due to trauma or ischaemic cardiac pain.

STOP

Reflect on a variety clinical situations and consider whether the timing of reassessment was appropriate.

What should be assessed?

The following issues should be considered when assessing pain:

- location and radiation
- intensity
- description/quality
- onset and duration
- aggravating and relieving factors.

Identifying the location and any radiation of pain is key to enabling diagnosis of the cause. There may be several sources all of which will need to be assessed and documented (Horgas, 2003). The intensity of the pain is used to determine the type of analgesia or treatment strategy (World Health Organization, 1986). A description of the quality of the pain may enable the cause to be identified, ie. somatic, visceral or neuropathic pain. Consideration of the onset, duration and variations of pain will aid diagnosis and planning of analgesic strategies.

Factors that cause or increase pain should be identified in order to plan analgesia administration, such as before physiotherapy. Some patients with persistent pain may have developed non-pharmacological strategies to relieve their pain, eg. distraction, position change. These must be assessed carefully and their continued use encouraged (McCaffery and Pasero, 1999).

Case studies

Patient A complains of sudden onset of severe crushing chest pain, with radiation into the left arm and jaw. The pain is worse on walking and is relieved by rest.
These symptoms may be indicative of ischaemic cardiac pain (angina), thus a detailed assessment not only aids diagnosis but also assists in choice of treatment strategy, eg. glyceryl trinitrate (GTN) spray, oxygen therapy.

Patient B complains of sudden onset severe lower back ache, with intermittent shooting pain from the left buttock down the back of the left leg. Pain is worse on sitting or bending. Some relief is achieved with massage and walking.
These symptoms may be indicative of musculoskeletal injury with sciatic nerve involvement due to inflammation. Treatment may take the form of simple analgesics, including anti-inflammatory drugs. Non-pharmacological strategies, such as a heat pad or transcutaneous electrical nerve stimulation (TENS), may also be considered. The patient should be discouraged from sitting for long periods of time or from lying on a hard surface, as immobility may lead to stiffening and muscle spasm. Gentle exercise (ie. walking or swimming) can be encouraged as and when simple analgesia relieves the pain.

Pain assessment tools

There are a number of pain assessment tools that are widely used in clinical practice. It is not possible to include all the tools that have been reported in the literature, therefore the most commonly used tools are described.

Verbal rating (categorical) scales, visual analogue scales (VAS) and numerical rating scales (NRS) have all been found to be valid and reliable for clinical use (Williamson and Hoggart, 2005). However, no one tool has been found to be reliable and valid for all patient populations. Therefore selection of the pain assessment tool should be based on the individual patient's needs and/or the specific population (Bird, 2003).

Unidimensional tools

Unidimensional tools include numerical rating scales and visual analogue scales.

The VAS for assessing pain consists of a 10cm line which has anchor statements at either end of the scale, 'no pain' and 'worst pain imaginable'. Patients are asked to indicate a point along the line that represents their pain severity. The NRS similarly has two anchor statements but can be used both verbally and visually. The NRS and the VAS are sensitive to changes in pain intensity. However they require careful explanation and presentation to ensure patient comprehension. Visual impairment may limit the usefulness of the VAS tool. Both these tools lend themselves to cross-cultural use/translation, although in the case of the NRS the patient needs to be able to comprehend pain as a number.

Numerical rating scale

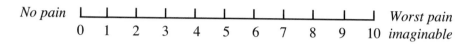

No pain   0   1   2   3   4   5   6   7   8   9   10   *Worst pain imaginable*

Visual analogue scale

No pain —————————————————————————— *Worst pain imaginable*

Categorical scales

Categorical scales can be verbally administered (VRS) and are associated with high completion rates as they are quick and simple to use. They require minimal training and lend themselves to translation for multicultural use. However, they are less sensitive than a VAS or an NRS and may be subject to bias.

0 = no pain   1 = mild pain   2 = moderate pain   3 = severe pain

Picture scales

A series of faces (usually four or five) depicting various expressions ranging from very happy to very distressed are shown to the patient (see *Figure 3.1*). Facial expressions are often assigned a category or numerical value. Patients are asked to point to the face that depicts the intensity of their pain. The Faces Scale is easy to use and is suitable for children, multicultural use and for older patients, although visual difficulties may prevent completion (Bird, 2003).

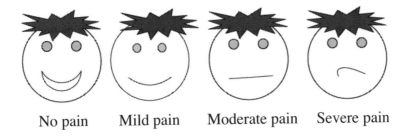

No pain   Mild pain   Moderate pain   Severe pain

Figure 3.1: The Faces Scale.

Multidimensional tools

A number of multidimensional tools have been developed to assess pain. The most widely validated tool in research and practice is the McGill Pain Questionnaire (Herr and Mobily, 1991). However, while these tools are useful for the assessment of persistent pain they can prove lengthy and inappropriate in many acute settings. The Short-form McGill Pain Questionnaire takes about five minutes to complete and is suitable for assessing the multidimensional nature of acute pain (Melzack, 1987). It consists of three indices:

- A total of 15 descriptors (11 sensory, 4 affective) are ranked on a categorical scale of none, mild, moderate, severe.
- A visual analogue scale.
- A present pain intensity scale (PPIS).

The 11 sensory descriptors in the short-form McGill Pain Questionnaire are: aching, burning, tender, throbbing, stabbing, heavy, gnawing, sharp, splitting, cramping and shooting.

Body charts

Body charts (*Figure 3.2*) showing part or the whole of the body are useful for documenting pain sites, but require the patient to have fine motor movement, co-ordination and visual integrity (Rowlingson, 1994).

Observation of behaviour and physiological responses

The accuracy of pain assessment through observation of a patient's behaviour and vital signs is inferior to self-report (Beyer *et al*, 1990). However, in some circumstances self-report is not feasible. Therefore in patients under the influence of anaesthetics or sedation, without adequate verbal skills or who are cognitively

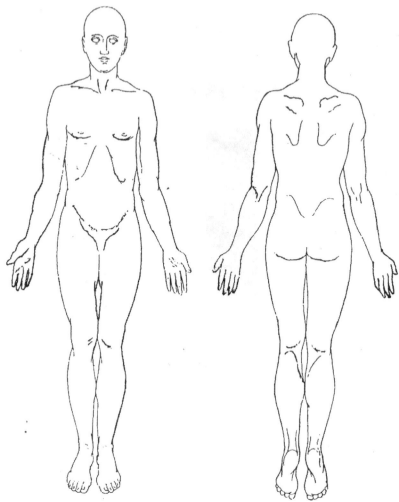

Figure 3.2: Example of a body chart.

impaired, the intensity of pain can only be estimated from the patient's behavioural and physiological responses. When assessing pain in people with severe cognitive impairment family members and carers also have an important role in providing information on expression and associated behaviours.

Visual displays of pain include:

- grimacing
- agitation or aggression
- restlessness/irritability
- withdrawal
- lying rigid in the bed
- pallor, sweating, nausea and/or vomiting.

Physical signs include:

- hypertension
- tachycardia
- muscle splinting or spasm around the pain site
- pallor
- sweating
- dilated pupils
- anxiety, fear, loss of sleep, and fatigue
- increased heart and respiratory rate.

Choosing a pain assessment tool

When selecting a pain assessment tool it is important to consider the following:

- It must be appropriate to the setting and the type of pain experience.
- The simpler it is the better.
- It must be easy for patients to use/understand.
- It needs to be consistent.
- Health care professionals need to re-evaluate/record.
- Health care professionals need to be willing to change treatment if it is not working.

STOP
Reflect on the pain assessment tools that you have seen in various clinical settings. Were they appropriate for the patient group?

Documentation

Documentation formalises the pain assessment process, promotes multidisciplinary communication between those caring for people over a 24-hour period and has legal implications (Paice *et al*, 1995). The results of any assessment should be documented in the nursing records, a specific pain assessment chart, or included as part of a routine observation chart.

Conclusion

Accurate assessment of acute pain is a prerequisite to diagnosing the cause and in ensuring appropriate treatment of pain. The choice of pain assessment tool will depend on the situation but it is essential that the tool is reliable and valid, and, to ensure continuity of care, consistent.

Health care workers must not allow their personal beliefs or biases to override the patient's self-report. Consider this: accepting and responding to the patient's report of pain will occasionally result in analgesics being given to some patients who are addicted or malingering. However, doing so ensures that everyone who has pain receives the best possible pain management. Accepting this will ensure that you never fail to help those who are in pain and therefore no one can find fault with your behaviour or professional conduct (Pasero and McCaffery, 2001).

Implications for nursing practice

- Pain will not be treated effectively unless it is assessed accurately.
- Effective communication in a trusting nurse–patient relationship is essential to help people express their pain.
- The results of any assessment should be documented in the nursing records, using a specific pain assessment chart.
- Nurses must not allow their personal beliefs to override the patient's self-report.

Key points

- Failure to undertake assessment of the individual's pain experience may lead to misdiagnosis and inappropriate or inadequate treatment of pain.
- The most effective way of measuring the amount of pain a person experiences is self-report. The accuracy of pain assessment through observation of a patient's behaviour is inferior to self-report.
- Pain should be assessed on admission to hospital or at a pre-assessment clinic in order to establish a baseline and information about how an individual usually copes with pain.
- There are a number of pain assessment tools that are widely used in practice.
- Documentation formalises the pain assessment process.

References

Beyer JE, McGrath PJ, Berde CB (1990) Discordance between self-report and behavioural pain measures in children age 3-7 years after surgery. *J Pain Sympt Manag* **5**: 350–6.

Bird J (2003) Selection of pain measurement tools. *Nursing Standard* **18**(13): 33–9.

Briggs M, Dean KL (1998) A qualitative analysis of nursing documentation of post-operative pain management. *J Clin Nurs* **7**: 155–63.

Closs S (1994) Pain in the elderly: A neglected phenomenon? *J Adv Nurs* **19**(6): 1072–81.

Cousins M, Power I (1999) Acute and post-operative pain. In P Wall, R Melzack (Eds.) *The Textbook of Pain* (4th edn.) Churchill Livingstone: Edinburgh.

Hamill R (1994) The physiologic and metabolic response to pain and stress. In R Hamill, J Rowlingson (Eds.) *Handbook of Critical Care Pain Management*. McGraw-Hill: New York.

Herr K, Mobily P (1991) Complexities of pain assessment in the elderly: Clinical considerations. *J Gerontol Nurs* **17**(4): 12–19.

Horgas A (2003) Pain management in elderly adults. *J Infusion Nurs* **26**(3):161–5.

Melzack R (1987) The short form McGill Pain Questionnaire. *Pain* **30**: 191–7.

McCaffery M, Pasero C. (1999) *Pain: Clinical Manual* (2nd edn.) Mosby: St Louis, MO.

Paice J, Mahon SM, Faut-Callahan M (1995) Pain control in hospitalized postsurgical patients. *Medsurg Nursing* **4**: 367–78.

Pasero C, McCaffery M (2001) The patient's report of pain: Believing vs. accepting. There's a big difference. *Amer J Nurs* **101**(12): 73–4.

Rowlingson J (1994) The assessment of pain in the critically ill. In K Puntillo (Ed.) *Pain in the Critically Ill: Assessment and Management*. Aspen: Philadelphia PA.

Seers K (1987) Perceptions of pain. *Nurs Times* **2**: 37–42.

Watt-Watson J (1987) Nurses' knowledge of pain issues: A survey. *J Pain Sympt Manag* **2**: 207–11.

Williamson A, Hoggart B (2005). A review of three commonly used pain rating scales. *J Clin Nurs* **14**(7): 798–804.

World Health Organisation (1986) *Cancer Pain Relief*. WHO: Geneva

CHAPTER 4

The management of acute pain

Angela Roberts

What is acute pain?

Acute pain is pain of sudden onset but limited duration and there is usually a relationship between the pain and disease or injury (Ready and Edwards, 1992). The International Association for the Study of Pain (IASP) defines pain as an 'emotional and sensory experience associated with actual or potential tissue damage and expressed in terms of such damage' (Merskey, 1979), and it is increasingly becoming recognised that acute and chronic pain may represent a continuum of pain rather than two separate entities.

The importance of managing acute pain effectively

It is understood that for patients to recover well from surgery or trauma they need to be able to breathe deeply and cough, and be able to move around as much as possible to prevent the formation of a deep vein thrombosis or chest infection, but what is less well understood is the need to treat acute pain effectively to prevent chronicity. When the body experiences a noxious (painful) stimulus, sensory information is conveyed to the brain via medium-diameter myelinated Aδ fibres and small-diameter slow conducting unmyelinated C fibres. The fibres convey this sensory information to nociceptor-specific areas within lamina I and II of the dorsal horn, and also to wide dynamic range neurones in lamina V. Information then passes via the spinothalamic tract to the thalamus and then on to the somatosensory cortex in the brain where perception of pain takes place. However, if there is intense sensory information travelling through the dorsal horn cells because the pain has not been treated effectively or is very severe, there is an increase in the action potential output from these dorsal horn cells, a condition know as 'wind up'. If left unchecked this can lead to central sensitisation and the possibility of patients going on to develop chronic pain conditions (Woolf and Salter, 2000).

STOP

List four reasons why it is important to treat acute pain swiftly and appropriately.

Different types of pain

Acute pain can be roughly categorised into nociceptive and neuropathic pain.

Nociceptive pain arises from tissue damage and is caused by trauma or surgery. It can be described by patients as a sharp, stabbing, aching, throbbing or dull pain and is often located around the area of tissue damage.

Neuropathic pain is associated with nerve damage, or altered neuronal firing within the nervous system. It is described by the IASP as 'pain initiated or caused by a primary lesion or dysfunction of the nervous system' (Merskey, 1994). Patients describe this pain as a burning shooting pain, or a pins and needles sensation following the tract of the damaged nerve. Both require different forms of analgesia to be effective.

Patients can also complain of spasm pain, especially following colorectal or orthopaedic surgery, and this is treated most effectively with an anti-spasmodic such as buscopan, baclofen or diazepam.

Drug management of acute pain

Opiate management

The mainstay of drug management for moderate to severe acute pain is opiate analgesia. The most common drug used is morphine; the standard opiate against which all the other opiates are compared. The main metabolite of morphine is morphine-6-glucuronide (M6G), a μ opioid agonist that produces analgesia. Derived from the poppy, morphine is very similar in chemical structure to natural morphine – the endorphins and encephalins produced by the body. Codeine is also a naturally occurring opiate produced from the poppy, and when taken into the body it is converted by the body to morphine. Not as strong as morphine, codeine is classified as a moderate opiate. Nine percent of the Caucasian population do not possess the gene to covert codeine to morphine and for these people codeine is not an effective analgesic (Caraco *et al*, 1996). Other opiates used are synthetic and mimic the properties of morphine and codeine. The most common of these are pethidine, fentanyl, oxycodone, tramadol and dihydrocodeine.

All these opiates work in the same way, by blocking the calcium channel at the synapse between the primary and secondary afferent neurones. All opiates are metabolised in the liver and excreted via the kidneys. Impaired renal function can result in a build up of the metabolite with an increased risk of side-effects. The most toxic metabolite is nor-pethidine the metabolite of pethidine, increased levels of which can lead to agitation, twitching and seizures (Simopoulos *et al*, 2002). For this reason the use of pethidine has been declining in recent years.

Common side-effects of opiates

All opiates have similar side-effects; the stronger the opiate the greater the risk. Respiratory depression is the side-effect that causes most concern among the medical profession; it is a potential problem because there are μ receptors in the brain. Regular monitoring of patients' respiratory rate is required when they are receiving strong opiates, and, if this becomes a problem, they should be treated with naloxone. Another side-effect is sedation, which can cause concern especially in the elderly, and is often a precursor to respiratory depression. Nausea and vomiting tend to be the biggest problem clinically. By their action on the chemoreceptor trigger zone opiates tend to make people nauseous, however, this is easily resolved by giving appropriate and regular anti-emetics. Pruritis can be a problem. It is caused by a histamine release in the body in response to receiving a foreign substance and can be treated effectively with anti-histamines. Constipation is a problem with stronger opiates and if their use is prolonged. There are opiate receptors in the bowel and opiates affect the peristaltic action of the gut. By regularly reviewing the strength of analgesia required and giving aperients if necessary this problem can be overcome.

Local anaesthetics in acute pain management

Local anaesthetics have a great role to play in acute pain management as they have the potential to provide very effective analgesia. However, their place is limited as no oral preparations are available, they are short acting and usually have to be given by continuous infusion, and they are quite toxic if given intravascularly. The most common local anaesthetics used are lidocaine and bupivacaine. Their mode of action is to block the action potential of the pain nerves by blocking the sodium channel (Serpell, 2003). This effect often causes areas of numbness and hence freedom from pain. They can be used for minor surgery and suturing in accident and emergency departments. They can be injected along a nerve root or into a plexus of nerves such as in femoral or sciatic nerve blocks for fractured neck of femur or brachial plexus nerve block for pancreatic pain. They are used inter-operatively for wound infiltration and especially following orthopaedic surgery to enhance postoperative pain management, and are often a component of epidural analgesia.

Local anaesthetics are increasingly being used prior to surgery. This pre-emptive analgesic effect is to block afferent input to the brain prior to the increased effects of surgery and minimise the risk of central sensitisation developing (Woolf and Chong, 1993). An example of this is femoral nerve block for elderly patients experiencing fractured neck of femur. Patients can be comfortable at rest but suffer excruciating pain on movement. Opiates offer little benefit for the intense pain on movement, and can lead to increased sedation and nausea. If there is to be some delay before patients can go to theatre, a femoral block maintained with a continuous infusion of local anaesthetic can be very effective and reduce morbidity in this group of patients. Ideally these would be initiated in the accident and emergency department.

Side-effects of local anaesthetics

Toxicity from local anaesthetics is related to the amount of drug given, with the central nervous system and the cardiovascular system being the most affected. Initial effects are tingling in the hands and arms or around the mouth, followed by sedation, convulsions and death (Covino, 1988). Regular monitoring of patients receiving local anaesthetic infusions, including regular checking of the infusion rate, are of primary importance in preventing these events.

Non-steroidal anti-inflammatory drugs (NSAIDs)

Both opioids and local anaesthetics provide analgesia by affecting the sensory pathways taking information to the brain. NSAIDs however work at the site of the pain. They inhibit the formation of cyclo-oxygenase and hence prostaglandin production. Prostaglandins sensitise peripheral nerve endings and amplify the effects of inflammatory mediators such as bradykinin (Cashman, 1996). NSAIDs help the pain by reducing this sensitising effect, but are less effective at dealing with nociceptive pain. NSAIDs are best used in combination with an opiate when treating moderate to severe pain. The most common NSAIDs used are diclofenac and ibuprofen.

It has been discovered in the last decade that cyclo-oxygenase exists in two forms: cyclo-oxygenase 1 (COX-1) and cyclo-oxygenase 2 (COX-2) (Needleman and Isakson, 1997). Aspirin and most NSAIDs inhibit both COX-1 and COX-2, however cyclo-oxygenase inhibitors highly specific for the COX-2 isozyme have now become available. These have the advantage over traditional NSAIDs of reducing the incidence of adverse events such as bleeding and gastrointestinal ulceration, especially of benefit when used to treat post-operative pain.

Contra-indications to the use of NSAIDs

NSAIDs should not be used in the following situations:

* pregnancy
* bleeding disorders
* acute peptic ulceration
* history of hypersensitivity to aspirin
* severe renal impairment
* severe hepatic disease
* elderly patients because of the reduced elimination capacity.

Side-effects of NSAIDs
Side-effects usually occur following long-term use, and include gastro-intestinal ulceration, renal impairment and impaired haemostasis.

Paracetamol

Paracetamol is a mild analgesic and antipyretic that has a synergistic effect with opiates enhancing its analgesic effect. For this reason paracetamol is often given in combination with a moderate opiate, such as co-codamol (codeine and paracetamol), co-dydromol (dihydrocodeine and paracetamol) and Tramacet (tramadol and paracetamol). Its precise mode of action is unknown, but is thought to involve central cyclo-oxygenase inhibition (Muth-Selbach *et al*, 1999). It can be given orally, rectally or intravenously. Hepatotoxicity can be fatal if overdose occurs, but in normal dose regimes it is safe and well tolerated by the majority of the population.

Entonox

Entonox is a gaseous mixture of 50% oxygen and 50% nitrous oxide which, when inhaled, has good analgesic properties. Used extensively in maternity and accident and emergency departments and by paramedics, it provides a good level of analgesia for moving patients or for short painful procedures. It can also be used on wards for moving patients, repositioning limbs, removing drains and dressing changes.

Entonox is self-administered from a clearly defined cylinder (blue with a white collar) via a demand valve, which the patient opens on inspiration and closes on exhalation. The gas can be delivered via a facemask or a special T-tube which the patient holds in the mouth. Respiratory effort greater than normal breathing is required to open the demand valve, so it is important to check that the patient can activate the system prior to any procedure or movement commencing. Entonox gas has a short duration of action; once the patient stops inhaling the gas its analgesic effect stops. If the procedure is going to be particularly painful, it is advisable to give a longer-lasting opiate, ie. oromorph, prior to commencement so that the patient will have some residual analgesia after the procedure has finished.

Although entonox provides good analgesia for short procedures, by its mode of action it causes expansion of the spaces that contain the gas, which can be a problem if the excess cannot escape. For this reason for patients who suffer from or who have experienced any of the following, its use is contra-indicated.

- pneumothorax
- air embolism
- decompression sickness
- recent underwater dive
- following air encephalography
- severe bullous emphysema
- myringoplasty
- gross abdominal distension
- head injuries with impaired consciousness
- intoxication
- maxillo-facial injuries
- patient non-compliance.

The ideal in managing acute pain

The ideal pain management strategy when using analgesia is to use a combination approach. Because opiates, local anaesthetics, NSAIDs and paracetamol all work on different parts of the pain modulatory process all can be given safely together. By giving drugs in combination less is often needed to achieve analgesia than if the drug were given on its own. This also reduces the incidence of side-effects. The dose of all analgesic drugs given needs to be titrated to individual patient need and administered via the most appropriate route.

Modalities for managing acute pain

Oral and rectal preparations

Oral analgesia is the most common route if patients are able to tolerate fluids. However there may be a delay between the administration and onset of analgesia due to the variability in rate of absorption, and the effect of first pass metabolism. To overcome this, sublingual, buccal and transmucosal preparations are available which allow for greater drug bioavailability as more enters the systemic circulation. The oral route is suitable for patients with mild to moderate acute pain.

Rectal preparations are also absorbed directly into the systemic circulation, giving greater bioavailability than the oral route, but the rate of absorption is very variable.

Parenteral preparations

With the parenteral route analgesia relates to the peak plasma concentration of the opiate. The subcutaneous route can be used for intermittent bolus doses or for continuous infusion, however the rate of absorption can be unpredictable. The intramuscular route is the most popular for patients in severe pain, or who cannot take oral preparations. However, absorption is erratic and there is great variability in the speed of onset, intensity of the analgesic effect and duration of its action. The intravascular route is referred to as the gold standard (Cashman, 2003) when rapid analgesia is required, as it has a rapid onset avoiding other routes of absorption. However the duration of the analgesic effect can be short-lived and intravenous infusions are required to maintain analgesia over a longer period of time. Because of the increased level of monitoring required when patients have continuous infusions of opiates these are often restricted to intensive care and high dependency units. To overcome the need for repeated intravascular injections, intravenous patient controlled analgesia (PCA) became available in the late 1970s and has revolutionised the way post-operative pain is now managed.

Patient controlled analgesia (PCA)

PCA is a technique that allows patients to administer their own analgesia via a programmable device. The analgesic used is usually morphine, but methadone, fentanyl and oxycodone are also used. The advantages are quality analgesia titrated to the patient's individual requirements enabling patients to comply better with physiotherapy and improve respiratory function, compared to intramuscular injections. The principle of PCA involves a dose of opiate on demand with a lockout interval usually of five minutes, the option of a background infusion, although rarely used in ward situations, and a one-hourly or four-hourly limit. Patients like the concept of being in control of their own analgesia, a strong psychological concept, and it avoids the clock watching of four-hourly intramuscular injections.

Contra-indications to PCA use are:

- Patient compliance: If patients are not cognitively aware or are unable physically to push the administration button, PCA is unsuitable.
- Lack of appropriately trained staff.

Monitoring of patients with PCA analgesia requires regular observations and documentation of pulse, blood pressure, respiratory rate and sedation level, pain scores at rest and on movement, and observation of the PCA device and total amount of analgesia given.

The amount of analgesia required by patients will vary depending upon the type of surgery or trauma they have undergone, and any other concomitant disease they have. As a general rule once patients are tolerating fluids, oral analgesia can be introduced and the PCA opiate discontinued once its use is minimal or it is no longer required.

Inhaled preparations

The lungs have a large surface area and as such provide a potential site for the absorption of inhaled analgesics (Cashman, 2003). However, there are very few drugs that have been found to be effective via this route. The most successful is entonox. The intranasal route can also be used with absorption through the nasal mucosa and intranasal diamorphine is successfully being used in some hospitals.

Topical preparations

If preparations are lipid soluble they can permeate the skin membrane and enter the blood circulation without first pass metabolism (Cashman, 2003). Some topical preparations are creams (NSAID gels or capsaicin cream) but most involve a transdermal delivery system, such as a patch. Of the opiates only fentanyl and temgesic are lipid soluble enough to be used effectively in this way, and analgesia is delivered at a controlled rate for a defined period of time usually three days. This method of delivery is not suitable for the treatment of acute pain as it does not allow for variable doses to be given. However, a new technique called iontophoresis causes electrically charged particles of a drug to be propelled through the skin by electrorepulsion (Cashman, 2003). Clinical trials using patient controlled patches are under way at present.

Epidural analgesia

Epidural analgesia is a means of providing potentially excellent pain relief. It is a technique whereby a catheter is inserted into the epidural space under strict sterile conditions, usually in an anaesthetic room prior to surgery. Through this catheter drugs can be infused continuously to provide analgesia. Drugs can be administered via a continuous infusion only or with a continuous infusion plus patient controlled bolus option, usually with a 30-minute lockout.

Opioids administered into the epidural space have been proven to provide prolonged segmental analgesia, with less systemic and central side-effects than when opioids are given systemically (Cousins and Mather, 1984). It is usual for fentanyl to be used as it is more lipophylic and binds to the fats in the epidural space although morphine, which is more hydrophilic, is used successfully in many hospitals. The use of epidural local anaesthetics, usually bupivacaine or levobupivacaine, provides advantages over opiates in that in blocking the sympathetic nerves epidural anaesthetics help reduce the stress response to surgery. Additionally, local anaesthetics do not inhibit bowel function in the same way as opiates (Liu *et al*, 1995). It is usual for a combination of an opiate and a local anaesthetic to be used. The advantage of combination drugs is the reduction in side-effects from giving the drugs on their own. This synergistic effect means lower doses of the drugs need to be given.

There are several advantages to using epidural analgesia. Compared to intravenous opiates and PCA, patients suffer fewer pulmonary complications and are better able to mobilise and comply with physiotherapy. Epidural analgesia causes less ileus and if used in conjunction with early feeding and mobilization has been shown to reduce hospital stay (Kehlet and Dahl, 1993). Epidural analgesia can be used effectively to treat:

- inter-operative pain
- post-operative pain
- traumatic pain
- obstetric pain
- chronic pain
- cancer pain.

Epidural analgesia is of benefit for any patient undergoing surgery where poorly controlled pain relief will cause detrimental effects. It has been found to be particularly beneficial for high-risk patients with cardiac or pulmonary insufficiency, and elderly patients undergoing major surgery.

STOP

Draw a diagram of the epidural space labelling what structures are above, below and to either side of the epidural space.

Contra-indications to epidural analgesia include the following:

- patient refusal
- inability to site the epidural due to spinal deformity
- altered coagulopathy
- shock or fixed cardiac output
- skin sepsis at the proposed site
- neurological disease or raised intra-cranial pressure.

Complications associated with epidural analgesia include dural puncture, which may occur during placement of the epidural catheter. Although the incidence is only 1%, if it is associated with dural puncture headache it can be distressing for patients (Giebler *et al*, 1997). Simple analgesia is the recommended treatment until the condition resolves. If it is severe a blood patch can be done but this does involve a further epidural to inject the blood.

Epidural haematoma or abscess formation are of particular concern as they can lead to compression of the spinal cord with resultant paralysis if not treated quickly. Although the incidence is low (less than 0.0007%) it does increase with the use of prophylactic anti-coagulation therapy (Rathmell *et al*, 2003). It is recommended that when low molecular weight heparin is used 12 hours should elapse before insertion or removal of an epidural catheter.

Some patients may develop neurological complications following epidural analgesia that persist, these include radicular pain, or spinal nerve root pain. Treatment is a full neurological assessment to rule out any other underlying cause followed by the administration of neuropathic agents such as gabapentin (Rathmell *et al*, 2003).

Side-effects of epidural analgesia

A range of side-effects are specific to opiates including pruritis, urinary retention, nausea and vomiting and respiratory depression.

Pruritis is more common in the epidural administration of opiates than with their systemic administration. However, it is still an uncommon side-effect and is dose related. It is more likely to be isolated to the face, neck and upper thorax and can be treated with antihistamines or low dose naloxone (Chaney, 1995).

It is difficult to establish the exact incidence of urinary retention as most patients are catheterised following major surgery. It is known that opioids can act at receptors in the sacral spinal cord affecting parasympathetic nervous system outflow. Local anaesthetics can also directly affect the parasympathetic nerves. Blockage of these nerves causes detrusor muscle relaxation and an increase in bladder capacity leading to urinary retention (Rawal *et al*, 1983).

Nausea and vomiting is thought to be caused by systemic absorption of the opioid in the epidural space, and also by cephaloid migration of the opioid into the cerebrospinal fluid and interaction with the opioid receptors in the area postrema (the vomiting centre) in the brain. Treatment is with anti-emetics (Rawal, 2003).

Respiratory depression may occur as a side-effect of opiates given by any route. It is of concern when opiates are delivered via the epidural route, especially if morphine is used, as there can be delay in onset. This is less common if fentanyl is used. Most of the opiate is absorbed via the epidural venous system and some will cross the dura and enter the cerebrospinal fluid. Although the risk of respiratory depression is less than 1% with epidural opiates regular monitoring of patients is vital to detect early occurrence (Rawal, 2003).

Specific side-effects of local anaesthetics include hypotension and sensory and motor loss. They can also cause vasodilation with resultant hypotension because of their effect on the blood circulation. This can be treated with colloid solutions such as gelofusin. However, other causes of hypotension need to be excluded such as hypovolaemia and bleeding.

The local anaesthetic action on the nerve roots in the spine can cause sensory and motor loss. Some sensory loss around the area of the wound will promote analgesia but sensory loss around the sacral area can lead to an increased risk of pressure ulcer formation. Motor loss in the legs will delay mobility and increase the risk of thromboembolus. If this is a problem the epidural rate can be reduced or an alternative method of analgesia sought (Rawal, 2003).

Monitoring patients with epidural analgesia

Regular monitoring of patients with epidural analgesia is vital to detect the development of any early complications. Most hospitals have guidelines and protocols for monitoring and treating complications. Monitoring will include regular assessment of pulse, blood pressure, respiratory rate and sedation level to observe for side-effects from the opiate, and assessment of sensory and motor function associated with the local anaesthetic.

Special considerations

Elderly patients

Managing acute pain in elderly patients can be complex as this group often has other concomitant diseases such as arthritis and heart disease, and they may already be taking several other medications, increasing the risk of drug interactions. Because of advances in surgical and anaesthetic techniques, older people are undergoing surgery that in the past would not have been attempted. With age, functional status may diminish and cognitive ability may be impaired, making modalities like patient controlled analgesia inappropriate, and assessment of pain more difficult. There is also the perception that older people do not feel pain as much as younger people because of demyelination of the pain nerves that can occur with age. There may also be age-related pharmacodynamic and pharmacokinetic issues, making side-effects of opiates more of a problem. There may be delayed hepatic clearance; the liver can decrease in size by 25–40% in elderly people with a resultant reduction in hepatic blood flow (Macintyre *et al*, 2003).

Because of these age-related problems there is sometimes a reluctance among medical staff to give opiates to elderly patients, or only to give them very sparingly. Following surgery it is important to treat the pain effectively, as chest infections, myocardial ischaemia, infarction and thromboembolic complications are all possible post-operative complications.

All interventions mentioned in this chapter for managing pain can be used in elderly people, although, as mentioned, if cognitive ability is impaired patient controlled analgesia may not be suitable. However dosing needs to be titrated slowly and starting doses are often lower than for younger patients.

Psychological management of acute pain

Psychological management of acute pain is centred around information giving and reassurance. Giving information in pre-admission clinics about how post-operative pain will be managed gives reassurance, aids patient compliance and helps with informed consent. Involving patients in their pain management plan helps their understanding of pain management strategies. Unrelieved pain can also alter a patient's perception of pain. Prolonged pain can increase anxiety levels, lead to sleep deprivation, instigate a sense of loss of control and a feeling of demoralisation. If patients have particular psychological problems following an acute pain episode, such as post-traumatic stress disorder, they can be referred to a clinical psychologist.

Conclusion

Acute pain needs to be treated quickly and aggressively to minimise the risk of central sensitisation developing. Adequate analgesia following surgery is vital if patients are to recover quickly and if the risk of complications is to be reduced. Analgesia that can be titrated by patients either via patient controlled analgesia or epidural systems allows them more control and an ability to have extra analgesia to aid mobility and physiotherapy.

The appropriate mechanism for delivering analgesia needs to be tailored to individual patient needs and patients using PCA or having epidural analgesia need to have constant monitoring to detect early any side-effects.

Implications for nursing practice

- Nurses have a key role in educating patients about the benefits of good pain control.
- The amount of analgesia required by patients will vary depending on the type of surgery or trauma they have undergone.
- Pain is what the patient says it is.
- Adequate analgesia following surgery is vital if patients are to recover quickly, it also helps to reduce the risk of complications.

Key points

- Unrelieved acute pain can lead to life-threatening complications.
- The main treatment for acute pain is opioid analgesia. This can be administered in various forms often determined by local guidelines or policies.
- Opiates have many side-effects and nurses need to be alert to them.
- The ideal strategy when using analgesia is to use a balanced approach. By giving a combination often less of a drug is needed to achieve analgesia.
- Patient controlled analgesia is a technique that allows patients to administer their own analgesia via a programmable device. It gives patients some control over their pain relief.
- Psychological management of acute pain is centred around information giving and reassurance.

References

Caraco Y, Sheller J, Wood A (1996) Pharmacogenetic determination of the effects of codeine and prediction of drug interactions. *J Pharmacol Exp Ther* **278**: 1165–74.

Cashman J (1996) The mechanism of action of NSAIDS in analgesia. *Drugs* **52**(Suppl. 5): 12–23.

Cashman J (2003) Routes of administration. In D Rowbotham, P Macintyre (Eds.) *Clinical Pain Management. Acute Pain.* Arnold: London.

Chaney M (1995) Side effects of intrathecal and epidural opioids. *Can J Anaes* **42**: 891 – 903

Cousins M, Mather L (1984) Intrathecal and epidural administration of opioids. *Anesthesiology* **61**: 276–310.

Covino B (1988) Clinical pharmacology of local anaesthetic agents. In M Cousins, P Bridenbaugh (Eds.) *Neural Blockade in Clinical Anaesthesia and Management of Pain.* (2nd edn.) Lippincott: Philadelphia.

Giebler R, Scherer R, Peters J (1997) Incidence of neurological complications related to thoracic epidural catheterisation. *Anesthesiology* **86**: 55–63.

Kehlet H, Dahl J (1993) The value of "multi-modal" or "balanced analgesia" in postoperative pain treatment. *Anes Anal* **77**: 1048–56.

Liu S, Carpenter R, Machey D (1995) Effects of perioperative analgesic technique on rate of recovery after colon surgery. *Anesthesiology* **83**: 757–65.

Macintyre P, Upton R, Ludbrook G (2003) Acute pain management in the elderly patient. In D Rowbotham, P Macintyre (Eds.) *Clinical Pain Management. Acute Pain.* Arnold: London.

Merskey H (1979) Pain terms: A list with definitions and notes on usage. Recommended by the subcommittee on Taxonomy. *Pain* **6**: 249–52.

Merskey H (1994) Logic truth and language in concepts of pain. *Qual Life Res* **3**(suppl 1): S69–76.

Muth-Selbach U, Tegeder I, Brune K, Geisslinger G (1999) Acetaminophen inhibits spinal prostaglandin E2 release after peripheral noxious stimulation. *Anesthesiology* **91**: 231–9.

Needleman P, Isakson P (1997) The discovery and function of COX-2. *J Rheumatol* **24**: 6–8.

Rathmell J, Neal J, Liu S (2003) Outcome measures in acute pain management. In D Rowbotham, P Macintyre (Eds.) *Clinical Pain Management. Acute Pain.* Arnold: London.

Rawal N, Mollefors K, Axelsson K (1983) An experimental study of urodynamic effects of epidural morphine and of naloxone reversal. *Anesth Anal* **62**: 641–7.

Rawal N (2003) Intraspinal opioids In D Rowbotham, P Macintyre (Eds.) *Clinical Pain Management. Acute Pain.* Arnold: London.

Ready L, Edwards W (1992) *Management of Acute Pain: A Practical Guide.* Taskforce on Acute Pain. IASP Publications: Seattle.

Serpell M (2003) Clinical Pharmacology – Local anaesthetics. In D Rowbotham, P Macintyre (Eds.) *Clinical Pain Management. Acute Pain.* Arnold: London.

Simopoulos T, Smith H, Peeters-Asdourian C (2002) Use of meperidine in patient-controlled analgesia and the development of a normeperidine toxic reaction. *Arch Surg* **137**: 84–8.

Woolf C, Chong M (1992) Pre-emptive analgesia – treating postoperative pain by preventing the establishment of central sensitisation. *Anesth Anal* **77**: 362–79.

Woolf C, Salter M (2000) Neuronal plasticity: Increasing the gain in pain. *Science* **288**: 1765–9.

CHAPTER 5

The assessment of chronic pain

Kimberley Tordoff

Introduction

Accurate pain assessment is a prerequisite of effective control and is an essential part of nursing the patient in pain. In the assessment process, the nurse gathers information from the patient that allows an understanding of the impact of the pain. This guides the nurse in planning and implementing strategies for care. Pain is never static and so assessment and evaluation are always ongoing.

What is chronic pain?

It is important to know that not all pain is the same, either in its origin or its perception. Pain may be acute or chronic, may arise from inflammation or trauma or be related to a secondary disease such as cancer or diabetes. In some cases it may be due to the malfunctioning of the nervous system (neuropathic pain) or have no known cause. Whatever the cause, we need to be mindful that pain can be modified by factors such as culture and background, the patient's beliefs about pain and previous pain experiences as well as psychological issues. As such, no pain assessment is ever complete without exploring these issues.

In 1986 the International Association for the Study of Pain (IASP), defined pain as 'an unpleasant sensory or emotional experience associated with actual or potential tissue damage, or described in terms of such damage'. Pain is the most common reason for patients to consult their doctor.

It is recognised that there are four separate elements to pain as a clinical phenomenon.

- First, the detection by special receptors (nociceptors) of actual tissue damage which results in the transmission of nerve messages to the central nervous system (CNS).
- Second, the perception of pain when these impulses reach the CNS.
- Third, suffering that is a mood generated by higher emotional brain centres in response to the pain.

▪ Fourth, outward behaviour to the pain and suffering such as crying, limping or seeking medical help.

Understanding these different components can lead to a better pain assessment and management strategy and so too the adoption of appropriate treatment.

Most importantly, as McCaffery (1983) says, 'Pain is what the patient says it is.'

Descriptors of pain

As there are different types of pain, the way in which it is initially assessed is crucial to its effective treatment. Pain may be described as nociceptive in origin (arising from the stimulation of pain receptors) or neuropathic (arising from the nervous system). In addition, its duration can be described as acute or chronic for short and long-lasting pain, respectively.

In making these distinctions, it should be recognised that pain is highly individual and totally subjective and will vary in intensity and sensation from person to person. This is reflected in the wide range of words that people use to describe, for example, backache. One person may use descriptors such as 'heavy, tiring and miserable' but another person will say 'stabbing, vicious and distressing'. The choice of words reflects the physical, psychological and social aspects of the pain as perceived by the individual (see *Table 5.1*).

This chapter addresses the assessment of chronic nociceptive and neuropathic pain. Acute pain is discussed in *Chapter 3*.

Chronic nociceptive pain

If pain after injury or surgery persists after the normal healing time, or it reoccurs over subsequent months or years, it will be classed as chronic. Such pain may also be due to diseases that interrupt normal tissue function, for example, arthritis.

Chronic neuropathic pain

Neuralgias and neuropathies are among the most difficult causes of chronic pain to understand and treat. Although very variable, the pain can be intense and very severe (post-herpetic neuralgia, trigeminal neuralgia). In other cases there may be constant aching, loss of sensation or shooting pains and tingling which can be equally distressing.

In some of the cases the cause can be traced to a disease such as diabetes which causes peripheral neuropathies or trauma that has caused nerve damage, but often a precise cause cannot be found.

Table 5.1: Words used by patients to describe pain

Aspect of pain	Descriptor
What it feels like	Flickering, pulsing, throbbing, beating, pricking, pounding, drilling, sharp, shooting, hot, searing, stinging, heavy, aching, itchy, rasping, dull, sore, crushing, pulling, cutting, pinching
How it affects mood	Desperate, tiring, exhausting, sickening, suffocating, fearful, terrifying, punishing, cruel, vicious, killing, wretched, blinding
Its character	Mild, annoying, discomforting, troublesome, distressing, miserable, severe, intense, horrible, excruciating, unbearable

Several categories of neuropathic pain exist.

- It may be mechanical due to trapped or compressed nerves. For example, slipped lumbar vertebrae or invasive tumours.
- It may be due to diseases such as diabetes or due to chronic malnutrition.
- Nerve changes following shingles can cause post-herpetic neuralgia.
- Phantom limb pain can occur post-amputation.
- Pain may arise for no apparent reason.

Pain with no apparent cause

Assessing and treating chronic pain for which there is no known cause is a challenging area. It can range from simple back pain to complicated facial pains and headaches. Although sometimes treatable, it often fails to respond well to medication and other therapies and can cause a serious reduction in the patient's quality of life.

Figure 5.1 illustrates the complex array of factors that influence the way people experience pain. We need to be mindful that while medication can affect some areas, skilled nursing can influence them all.

The assessment of pain

The initial assessment of pain is the start of a journey that the nurse makes with the patient, the destination being adequate pain control.

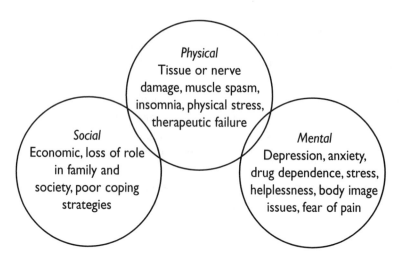

Figure 5.1: Some of the many factors that contribute to the concept of chronic pain.

The most critical factor to the successful treatment of pain, whether the pain is acute or chronic, is establishing a standard for assessing the existence and intensity of the pain. If the health care team does not have a standard for doing this then, quite simply, each person will carry out the whole process differently, resulting in poor pain control.

Research shows that most nurses tend to underestimate patents' pain (Zalon, 1993) or fail to assess it altogether. Donovan *et al* (1987) studied 353 patients on medical and surgical wards and found that less than half of them recalled being asked about the presence of pain. Nurses are not the only care givers who are remiss about this, a study by Grossman *et al* (1991) demonstrated that even experienced doctors can fail to appreciate the effects of moderate to severe pain.

The very nature of chronic pain means that it can be difficult to assess. Patients may present with more than one symptom, have pain in multiple places or else have other problems that they do not directly attribute to their pain but which are inextricably linked, for example, depression, sleep deprivation and nausea.

Changes in mood may alter the experience of pain quite dramatically (McCaffery and Beebe, 1989) and there are well-established links between chronic pain and depression (Gray, 2001). Therefore, chronic pain assessment needs to acknowledge these factors as well as others that will modulate pain sensitivity (see *Table 5.2*).

Practical pain assessment

Chronic pain assessment will most likely take the form of an informal interview that should be conversational in nature. As much information

Table 5.2: Factors relating to pain sensitivity

Sensitivity increased	Sensitivity decreased
Discomfort	Relief of symptoms
Insomnia	Sleep
Fatigue	Rest
Anxiety	Sympathy
Fear	Understanding
Anger	Companionship
Sadness	Diversional activity
Depression	Reduced anxiety
Boredom	Elevation in mood

as possible should be gathered about the pain without the interview being too time-consuming. The use of open and leading questions is helpful. General observation of the patient may be helpful with regard to wincing/grimacing, limping, the use of aids to help with walking and the patients' functional capacity.

Typical questions include:

- Tell me about your pain.
- Can you show me where you have pain?
- What makes the pain worse?
- What makes the pain better?
- Is the pain constant?
- Are there any times of the day when you are pain free?
- Can you tell me any words that describe the pain? [You may need to suggest a few].
- How much [in a percentage] do your painkillers reduce your pain?
- Does the pain go anywhere else? [Radiation].
- Does the pain disturb your sleep?
- Do you understand what is causing your pain?

Assessment of location

Location can be assessed using a human body chart (see *p. 32*). Patients are asked to shade in the areas where they experience pain. Body charts are particularly useful with patients who have more than one area of pain. They provide a useful record of the site and distribution of the pain, and the percentage of body surface involved can be measured.

Pain assessment tools

The use of pain assessment tools increases the effectiveness of nursing interventions and also helps to improve the standard of pain control that patients receive. They can enable pain to be monitored regularly (Twycross *et al,* 1996) and improve communication between staff and patients if used correctly (Raiman, 1986). Higginson (1998) suggests that taking assessments directly from the patient is the most valid way of collecting information. Encouraging patients to take an active role by using pain assessment charts can help to increase their confidence and make them feel involved in their care.

However, some caution needs to be exercised with the use of pain charts and assessment tools. The correct tool needs to be used if it is to be valid, and pain assessment charts need to be completed correctly and at regular intervals. Some tools focus on the intensity of the pain and are more suited to the assessment of acute pain. With chronic pain it is necessary to use a tool that also assesses the impact on the patient's psychosocial needs, or at least considers them.

Hancock (1996) recommends that pain assessment tools should meet the following criteria:

- Simplicity: They are easy to understand for all the patients.
- Reliability: Results can be reproduced when used in similar patient groups.
- Sensitivity: The tool is sensitive to the patient's pain.
- Accuracy: There is little room left for error.
- Practical: The tool is easy to use for patients and staff.

STOP
Read up on three pain assessment tools and find one that may be appropriate for the area that you are working in. If a pain assessment tool is in regular use discuss the pros and cons of it with your mentor, it may not be the right one.

Assessment of intensity

Pain rating scales (see *Chapter 3*) are often used in order to quantify the patient's pain experience, the simplest of these being visual analogue scales (VAS), numerical rating scales (NRS) and verbal rating scales (VRS). A more representative assessment of the patients' pain can be made with a pain diary.

Visual analogue scales
Visual analogue scales comprise a 10cm line with no pain at the left end and worst pain imaginable at the right end. Patients are then asked to make a mark on the line that best represents their pain intensity and the measurement is

taken in centimetres from the left end to the mark to give a pain score. Some patients find this scale difficult to conceptualise and their scores can be an inaccurate reflection.

Numerical rating scales

Numerical rating scales involve asking patients to rate their pain on a scale of 0 to 100, giving 101 possible answers, or 0 to 10, giving 11 possible answers. These tools are simple enough for most people to use and not prone to much measurement error.

Verbal rating scales

In verbal rating scales patients are requested to indicate which word best describes their pain from the list below:

- none
- mild
- moderate
- severe
- excruciating.

Each category is then assigned a numerical value if analysis is required (0, 1, 2, 3, and 4). One criticism of this scale is that it is relatively insensitive due to the small number of categories.

It is important to remember that pain scales give an indication of how the patient's pain is and they are only useful if they are used regularly and the results documented and acted upon. It is important to try to get information about the patient's pain on movement as well as at rest and to find out what level of pain the patient would feel was acceptable. This is very important as both the patient and the health care team need to be aiming for the same goal.

Pain diaries

Pain diaries provide detailed information on the nature of the pain, when it occurs and its severity, as well as the efficacy of medications or interventions taken. Pain can be rated several times during the day or at the end of it as an average score. Medications and their effectiveness can also be recorded, as well as the patient's activity level and mood.

Quality of the pain

As discussed earlier different types of pain have different qualities and by assessing the nature of the pain the treatment will be more appropriate. A deep knife-like pain or aching inside is indicative of visceral pain. Burning, stabbing, shooting and electric type of pain may be neuropathic. Musculoskeletal pain can manifest as aching, throbbing, and gnawing that is worse with movement and at the start or end of the day.

The patient may have difficulty explaining the quality of the pain and so the nurse needs to have knowledge of the common descriptors outlined in *Table 5.1*.

Remember that other members of the team may have assessed the patient's pain, for example the physiotherapist. Findings should be discussed with them as it may give more information from a different perspective.

Misconceptions about pain

Probably the most challenging aspect of caring for a patient in pain is to accept that the sensation of pain is completely subjective. The 1983 definition from Margo McCaffery that 'pain is whatever the experiencing person says it is, existing whenever he says it does' is still valid. In recent years other statements have endorsed that of McCaffery, for example, 'the mainstay of pain assessment is the patient's self-report' (Jacox *et al*, 1994). However, almost all of us at some time will discount a patient's report of pain. It is therefore important that we are aware of the many misconceptions surrounding pain that may cause us to doubt a patient. This will help us to:

- Identify our professional responsibility to the patient regarding duty of care.
- Prevent us from acting on our misconceptions.
- Educate others to examine their reasons for not believing a patient's report of pain.

A list of common misconceptions and how they can be corrected is given in *Table 5.3*. Pain assessment in relation to the NMC Code of Professional Conduct is given in *Table 5.4*.

STOP
Reflect on some of the patients in pain that you have nursed. Have you always believed that their pain is real and acted accordingly? Have you ever worked with nurses and doctors who have not believed the patient's pain? How did that make you feel? What will you do next time you come across these kinds of misconceptions?

Case study

Ted is a 35-year-old builder who is covered in tattoos, some of them offensive. Despite his looks he is a polite and honest man with a quiet disposition. He was diagnosed with chronic pancreatitis 2 years ago and since then has become diabetic due to his pancreatic insufficiency. He is frequently admitted to hospital due to his brittle diabetes and his pain.

Table 5.3: Common misconceptions about pain

Misconception	Correction
You can teach patients to tolerate pain, the longer they have pain the more used to it they become	Tolerance to pain is an individual response; people with prolonged pain tend to have a lower threshold to it
Personal beliefs are fundamental in assessing pain	This does not constitute a professional approach to assessing a patient's pain. The patient's credibility is not the issue
Nurses and doctors are the authority on the nature and existence of pain	The gold standard for assessing and reporting pain is the patient. There is nobody else who can experience the sensation of that pain
Lying about the existence of pain, or malingering is common	Very few people lie about the existence of pain and fabrication about pain is very rare
Visible signs accompany pain and can be used to verify how severe it is	Lack of pain expression does not mean lack of pain. Humans have the ability to adapt to situations and so patients with chronic pain have the ability to carry on almost as normal
Patients should not be given painkillers until a reason for the pain is diagnosed	Pain should be treated even if the cause is not known. Patients have the right to have their pain treated and their reports of pain accepted and acted upon

Over the last 2 years he has become more despondent with his admissions as the staff tend to think that he is drug seeking and do not believe his pain is as bad as he reports, despite his proven pathology. Ted is refusing to be admitted into hospital when his GP wishes it, as he says his pain will be better controlled at home as he can take the medication he needs when he requires it rather than asking the nurses, who 'can take hours'.

What are the issues that need addressing and how could you deal with them?

Table 5.4: Pain assesment in relation to the NMC Code of Professional Conduct

Respect the patient as an individual	If one assessment/intervention is not appropriate try another
Promote a partnership in care	Patients need to be involved in decision making
Promote dignity and respect	Pain control is a basic human right
Obtain consent prior to treatment	Ensure that the patient understands what you are going to do and why
Maintain professional knowledge and competence	Ensure that you are experienced and sufficiently well-trained to do what you are required. If not ask for guidance
Keep accurate records	Vital to assess and re-evaluate the patient; this is also a legal requirement

Beliefs about pain control and patients' rights

Nurses' beliefs about pain relief and patients' rights form the foundation of suggested approaches to the adequate assessment and treatment of patients in pain.

Pain control should:

- Rank highly on the list of nursing priorities for patient care.
- Be a legitimate therapeutic goal.
- Be patient-controlled, ie. patients are the authority on the assessment of their pain.

Patients have the right to:

- Decide the intensity of pain that they are willing to tolerate.
- Be informed of all possible methods of pain relief as well as the possible outcomes of those treatments, and be allowed to choose which of those treatments they wish to pursue.

It should also be recognised that the health care team has the right to refuse a treatment that it deems may be harmful to a patient.

STOP

Find out if the area in which you are working is covered by the acute or chronic pain team. Make enquiries to see if you can spend some time working with them.

Implications for nursing practice

- The initial assessment of pain is the start of a journey that the nurse makes with the patient, the destination being adequate pain control.
- Most nurses tend to underestimate patients' pain.
- The use of a pain assessment tool has been shown to increase the effectiveness of nursing interventions and also to improve the standard of pain control that patients receive.
- Accurate pain assessment is an essential part of nursing the patient in pain.
- A multidisciplinary approach is the best model.

Key points

- Pain is never static and so assessment and evaluation are always ongoing.
- Not all pain is the same, either in its origin or its perception.
- Pain is a highly individual and totally personal experience. The intensity and sensation will vary from person to person.
- The very nature of chronic pain means that it can be difficult to assess.
- Chronic pain assessment needs to acknowledge a number of descriptors including mood, depression and fatigue.

References

Donovan M, Dillon P, McGuire l (1987) Incidence and characteristics of pain in a sample of medical-surgical inpatients. *Pain* **30**: 69–78.

Gray E (2001) Linking chronic pain and depression. *Nurs Stand*, 15 (25), 33–6.

Grossman S, Sheidler V, Sweeden K *et al.* (1991) Correlation of patient and caregiver ratings of cancer pain. *J Pain Sympt Manag* **6**: 53-57.

Hancock H (1996) The complexity of pain assessment and management in the first 24 hours after cardiac surgery: Implications for nurses. Part 2. *Intensive Crit Care Nurs* **12** (5): 295–302.

Higginson I (1998) Can professionals improve their assessment? *J Pain Sympt Manag* **15**(3): 149–50.

International Association for the Study of Pain (1986) *Classification of Chronic Pain. Descriptions of Chronic Pain.* International Association for the Study of Pain: Seattle, WA.

Jacox A, Carr DB, Payne R *et al.* (1994) *Management of Cancer Pain: Adults' Quick Reference Guide.* Agency for Health Policy and Research: Rockville, MD.

McCaffery M (1983) *Nursing Management of the Patient in Pain.* JB Lippincott Co., Philadelphia.

McCaffery M, Beebe. A (1989) *Pain: Clinical Manual for Nursing Practice.* St. Louis, MO: C. V. Mosby.

Raiman J (1886) Pain relief: A two-way process. *Nursing Times* **82**(15): 24–8.

Twycross R, Harcourt J, Bergl S (1996) A survey of pain in patients with advanced cancer. *J Sympt Pain Manag* **12**(5), 273–82.

Zalon M (1993) Nurses. assessment of post-operative pain. *Pain* **54**: 329–34.

Useful websites

www.britishpainsociety.org
www.stopPain.org
www.blackwellroyalmarsdenmanual.com
www.painfoundation.org

CHAPTER 6

The management of chronic non-malignant pain

Lorraine Stevens

What is chronic pain?

Chronic pain can have a devastating effect on a person's life. It is a very personal sensation that cannot be seen by an observer and is difficult to describe to others. The International Association for the Study of Pain (1986) defines pain as 'an unpleasant sensory and emotional experience associated with actual or potential tissue damage, or described in terms of such damage'.

If pain after surgery or injury persists after the normal healing time, or if it reoccurs in the following months or even years it is classed as chronic pain.

Chronic pain is pain that is persistent in nature, and for which, in many cases, the underlying cause cannot be cured. Chronic pain may be due to a long-term incurable medical condition or disease, or it may have no obvious precipitating cause. There are differences in opinion among experts of how long you have to have pain before it is classed as chronic. However, most agree pain is chronic when it continues for longer than three months.

While acute pain serves a purpose and is a normal sensation that alerts the sufferer to a possible injury, chronic pain is different as the pain persists for weeks, months and sometimes years. Unlike acute pain chronic pain serves no purpose, as it does not act as a warning to the patient.

The patient may suffer an initial injury such as a back strain or an infection, where pain signals are triggered but, due to complex pain mechanisms, instead of the pain resolving it continues long-term.

There may be an ongoing cause for chronic pain such as arthritis; however, in many cases there may be no evidence of injury. This can lead to professionals not believing patients' reports of pain, leading to under-treatment or even non-treatment of the pain. There is a common misconception that patients lie about their pain. This is rare.

Is the problem widespread?

Unfortunately chronic pain is a worldwide problem. It affects millions of people and remains under-treated despite the availability of treatments.

Recent research confirms the magnitude of chronic pain as a major health problem throughout Europe. It is a burden to both the patient and society. Systematic reviews of studies on the prevalence of chronic pain show that in Europe 11–55% of the population is suffering with long-term non-cancer pain. (Breivik, 2003). It is one of the most common reasons why patients visit their general practitioner.

Physical and psychosocial problems

The non-treatment or under-treatment of chronic pain can have serious outcomes, including emotional, social and, importantly, physical effects. Chronic pain increases stress and causes problems with appetite and sleep. Psychological problems such as feelings of low self-esteem, powerlessness and depression frequently occur.

Common chronic complaints include low back pain, headache, arthritis, and neuropathic pain resulting from damage to nerves following surgery or injury. Unfortunately, even with currently available technology it remains difficult to diagnose the precise mechanisms and location of many types of chronic pain.

It has long been noted that chronic pain is under-treated. Without treatment, patients can spiral into a vicious circle of physical, social and emotional problems. In 2004 the Pain Society and the Royal College of General Practitioners endorsed five pledges to help people living with chronic pain. These pledges stated that there should be:

- Active involvement in the management of all people with persistent pain.
- Timely assessment of the patient's pain.
- Access to appropriate management and support.
- Access to relevant information.
- Access to adequate resources and facilitates.

Types of chronic pain

In order to treat the pain appropriately it is important to differentiate between the different types of pain. Effective treatment is achieved by careful and methodical assessment of symptoms. It is vital to remember that pain is what the experiencing person says it is, existing whenever he or she says it does (McCaffery, 1983). If patients report pain nurses should have no reason to think that they feel otherwise.

There are three main types of pain that derive from different areas of the body. Depending on the type of pain, patients will require different medications. This is why it is vital to diagnose the type of pain in order to treat it appropriately.

Musculoskeletal pain

Musculoskeletal pain is described as aching, throbbing or gnawing and occurs on activity. Examples of musculosketal pain include chronic low back pain, rheumatoid or osteoarthritis and fibromyalgia.

Visceral pain

Visceral pain arises from the internal (visceral) organs. It is described as a dull, sickening, aching pain. Examples of visceral pain include pancreatitis, angina and renal pain.

Neuropathic pain

Neuropathic pain is transmitted by a nervous system damaged either centrally or peripherally. It is described as shooting, burning or pins and needles. Examples of neuropathic pain include post-herpatic neuralgia, diabetic neuropathy and scar pain.

Assessment of chronic pain

Before a treatment plan can be formulated it is essential that an accurate assessment is undertaken. The very nature of chronic pain means that it can be difficult to assess. Pain is a subjective, complex and multifaceted experience and the initial assessment needs to gather as much information as possible about the nature, intensity, location and the effects that the pain has on the person's life. Many patients will have tried a plethora of treatments with limited success. The assessment needs to gather information about such treatments and establish why the patient thinks they were unsuccessful in order to avoid trying treatments that have failed in the past.

The multidisciplinary team approach

Chronic pain is very complex and involves many different problems. It can lead to disability, suffering and unrealised potential. Patients often become inactive or they over-work some days until their pain is so severe that they have to rest the next day. They become easily depressed and start to feel negative about themselves.

Remember the IASP definition tells us that pain has an emotional and sensory component. Treatments for chronic pain should reflect this. The main goal of the management of chronic non-cancer pain is to improve the patient's function while decreasing the frequency and the intensity of the pain, with an equal emphasis on both.

The approach should involve a multidisciplinary team to help patients to reduce their disability, challenge negative thoughts, and assist them to plan and pace their activities on a daily basis.

The team should include doctors, specialist nurses, physiotherapists, psychologists and occupational therapists.

STOP

What range of treatment approaches are available for the management of chronic pain?

There are several approaches to pain management, many of which can be used together. Most patients will have tried some or all of the following treatments.

- medication
- nerve block
- transcutaneous electrical nerve stimulation (TENS)
- physiotherapy
- surgery
- complementary therapies
- osteopathy, chiropractic and manipulation
- various psychological and behavioural training
- spinal cord stimulation.

Medication

The starting point of pain management should be based on the principle of the World Health Organization (WHO) ladder (see *Chapter 2*). Originally designed for use in cancer patients, it offers basic guidance for the effective management of pain.

The principle is that patients start on the first rung of the ladder with simple analgesia then, if the pain is not relieved and is moderate in intensity, they proceed to the next step and finally onto the third step if they are experiencing severe pain.

Assessment will reveal the degree of pain the patient is experiencing. Most patients on presentation will already have tried most of the analgesics in step one so will start at step two and proceed upwards as required.

Step one medications include non-opioid analgesics, aspirin, paracetamol, ibuprofen and diclofenac. Step two medications are weak opioids, such as dihydrocodeine, tramadol, co-codamol and co-proxamol. Step three medications are strong opioids, such as morphine, oxycodone, fentanyl and hydromorphone.

Adjuvant analgesia

At any of these steps the patient can be given adjuvant analgesia. Adjuvant analgesics are drugs that are primarily used for non-pain conditions but that have also been found to be useful analgesics. Examples of adjuvant analgesics include antidepressants, anticonvulsants, steroids, antispasmodics and benzodiazepines.

STOP

Amitriptyline, which was developed as an antidepressant, has been found to be very valuable for neuropathic pain. Using the above list and referring to the British National Formulary, name one drug in each of the other groups.

Using a preventive approach to the administration of analgesia

When administering medication it is important that the nurse maximises the effects of the analgesia used. To achieve this, analgesia must be given regularly. Along with regular doses, analgesia should be given 'as required', ie. for breakthrough pain, as soon as the pain begins. The pain should not be allowed to build up or it may require stronger doses to alleviate it. By giving analgesia regularly and as required, the patient will spend less time in pain and doses can be smaller than if the pain is allowed to increase. This will also help to reduce side-effects. Also, worry about the pain returning will reduce as will 'clock watching' behaviour, which occurs when patients are concerned about not obtaining pain relief when it is needed.

Titration of analgesia

It is important to adjust and individualise the dose for each patient as required, changing to the most appropriate route of administration, and choosing the drug that best suits the patient, ie. one with the lowest side-effects and greatest benefit.

The nurse's role

The relief of the patient's pain rests with the whole multidisciplinary team. However, it is the nurse who plays a key role in assuring good pain control. The nurse spends more time with the patient than any other health care professional and is in the best position constantly to reassess and evaluate the effectiveness of treatments.

The nurse's responsibilities include choosing the appropriate analgesia, determining whether to give it, evaluating its effectiveness and obtaining a change of prescription if needed.

See *Chapter 2* for a more detailed look at drug regimes and side-effects.

Nerve block

Nerve blocks are injections of local anaesthetic, steroids or neurolytic (chemical) agents, into or near the peripheral nerve, a sympathetic nerve plexus or a local trigger point. This procedure blocks nerve pathways in the spinal cord and prevents the brain from receiving messages so that the patient perceives less pain. They generally give short-term relief to allow mobilisation and return to normal activity. Nerve blocks tend to be part of the rehabilitation process and are rarely a cure. They can help many types of pain including low back pain with sciatica, neck pain, shoulder pain, post-herpetic neuralgia, complex regional pain syndromes, chronic pancreatitis and painful trigger points.

Types of nerve block include epidurals, joint injections, including ball and socket and facet joints, intercostal nerve block and sympathetic nerve block.

Side-effects are rare but include infection and allergic reaction. The steroids can produce fluctuations in blood sugar, fluid retention and increased blood pressure. The destruction of nervous tissue can produce loss of motor and sensory nerves.

Transcutaneous electrical nerve stimulation (TENS)

A TENS machine is a small battery-operated device that delivers rapid impulses of an electrical current to electrodes applied to the skin (see *Figure 6.1*). TENS machines normally have several settings and can give intense stimulation during periods of severe pain or a lower level background stimulation. Although effective for some individuals, TENS is only helpful when in use and the analgesic effect is not long-lasting. TENS machines are cheap, easy to use and lightweight and allow patients some control over their pain. Patients can alter the settings to increase or decrease the intensity depending on the level of pain. TENS feels like a tingling, buzzing sensation on the skin and is thought to work by closing the pain gates. Patients with pacemakers and who are early in pregnancy are contra-indicated.

Spinal cord stimulation

The use of stimulators in the spinal cord dates back to the 1960s. The 1980s saw improvements in patient selection, hardware and technical expertise and as a result this treatment modality grew in popularity. It is thought to be helpful in the treatment of neuropathic pain, ischaemic pain and refractory angina pectoris.

Treatment consists of percutaneous electrodes that are implanted in the epidural space and a current is passed between them from a battery-operated device. This method of treatment is expensive and so strict inclusion and exclusion criteria govern which patients receive it.

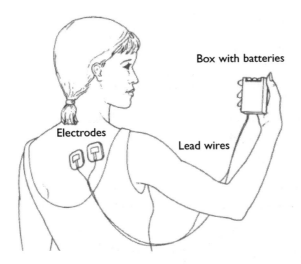

Figure 6.1: A Patient with a TENS machine.

Surgery

Surgery may be useful in some cases but its use in pain control is complex and details are beyond the scope of this chapter. Surgery can take many forms. For example, it can benefit patients suffering from certain pain syndromes, ie. trigeminal neuralgia and endometriosis.

Physiotherapy

Patients with chronic pain are often reluctant to mobilise the affected area due to increasing pain and fear of doing themselves more harm. The result is decreased mobility causing stiffness and what is commonly known as exaggerated pain behaviour.

Establishing a programme of physical exercise should be incorporated into any treatment plan. The benefits include increased mobility, decreased muscle strain and a reduction in muscle spasm. See *Chapter 9* for details of the different types of physiotherapy treatments available and their benefits.

Psychological and behavioural training

There is invariably a psychological component involved in most chronic pain, although, except in rare conditions, it is unlikely that psychological problems are the cause. However, they certainly affect the patient's ability to cope with pain. Many people who suffer chronic pain develop symptoms of depression, anxiety, loss of self-confidence, avoidance of activities and sleep disturbance.

Educational based programmes incorporating cognitive and behavioural therapies are useful in helping patients to come to terms with living with chronic pain. These are offered throughout the country at specialist pain clinics. Specific goals include:

■ Education to assist patients to manage their pain more effectively.
■ Relaxation.
■ Goal-setting and diversional methods.
■ Cognitive-behaviour training.
■ Stress management.

Because pain is such a uniquely personal experience, many people find these psychological techniques helpful. This subject is covered in more detail in *Chapter 10*.

Complementary therapies

Complementary therapies are becoming increasingly popular among patients with ongoing problems such as chronic pain. Patients often seek therapies to try to alleviate pain when traditional medicine has failed. There are a number of therapies available and it is difficult to define which method is helpful in which condition. The best advice is to use the therapy if the patient believes it helps. Unfortunately, there is little robust research to prove effectiveness of such therapies and so many treatments are not available on the National Health Service. The following treatments are available.

Relaxation

Chronic pain can cause a vicious circle of pain leading to tension, leading to further pain, as illustrated in *Figure 6.2*.

Often simple relaxation techniques can help patients relax and bring muscle tension under control and break the cycle. Relaxation and imagery are two simple techniques that may relieve tension and muscle spasm and may help to reduce chronic pain. Relaxation involves learning a series of breathing and muscle relaxation exercises. Relaxation can:

• help sleep and rest
• give a feeling of well-being
• lower blood pressure
• lower pulse rate
• lower temperature
• decrease muscle spasm
• reduce pain
• give a feeling of control over the situation.

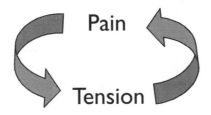

Figure 6.2: Pain causes tension which increases pain to form a pain-tension cycle.

Hypnosis/hypnotherapy

There is no single, accepted definition of hypnosis. Hypnosis is a broad concept and has been used for many different indications. Therapy with hypnosis (hypnotherapy) involves the use of many different techniques to induce deep relaxation. It is widely believed that all hypnosis is self-hypnosis (sometimes directed by another, ie. hypnotherapist) and that hypnotic thinking is a state of alertness and intense concentration, in fact similar to everyday thinking. Hypnotherapy does not involve loss of consciousness nor someone else controlling your mind. It is often used by psychologists in pain clinics to teach patients to manipulate their pain.

Acupuncture

The most widely used complementary therapy is acupuncture. It has risen in credibility since the 1990s and there has been some strong evidence for its use in dental pain, tennis elbow, low back pain, fibromyalgia, menstrual cramps and headaches. Acupuncture is now offered in most National Health Service pain clinics throughout Britain. Specialist nurses, doctors and physiotherapists are commonly trained to use acupuncture for musculoskeletal disorders.

The scientific basis for acupuncture is release of chemicals in the brain called endorphins that bind to the morphine receptors. This brings about altered sensation including analgesia. Magnetic resonance imaging (MRI) shows that acupuncture can decrease pain signals in some parts of the brain.

Acupuncture points are located in dermatomes, often a considerable distance from the pain. Many trigger points coincide with motor points in skeletal muscle. Needles are generally made of stainless steel. The length of the needle used and depth of penetration depends on the thickness of the underlying soft tissue. Needles may be inserted perpendicularly, obliquely or tangentially and are stimulated manually or with a mild electrical current.

Patients report feeling a sensation described as a deep, heavy, tingly warmth. Duration of treatment can range from 20 to 40 minutes and is commonly carried out in pain clinics or physiotherapy departments on a weekly basis. Frequency of treatment can be variable depending on the clinical problem and availability of resources. Although more studies are needed, the improvement in some patients appears to have a scientific basis.

Side-effects include bruising and infection at the needle site, fainting and nausea. Although it is generally safe there are risks involved and rupture of major vessels and organs has been reported.

Osteopathy and chiropractic

Osteopathy and chiropractic are manipulative therapies that work on the musculoskeletal system. Chiropractic focuses mainly on the spine and its effects on the nervous system. It claims to restore the spinal and musculoskeletal system to normal by using manipulative techniques and specific adjustment manipulating each joint in turn.

Reflexology

Reflexology is based on the idea that specific points on the feet and hands correspond to organs and tissues throughout the body. The practitioner applies pressure with fingers and thumbs on these points to treat a wide range of stress-related ailments.

Case study

Kate is a 54-year-old married woman who has worked as a nursing assistant in an old people's home for the past 20 years. She is a non-smoker, a social drinker and is overweight, weighing 75kg. When she is not working her lifestyle is fairly sedentary. She never exercises, claiming she is too busy.

While on duty she was helping an elderly lady back to her bed when the lady stumbled and fell to the ground. As Kate tried to prevent the fall she felt a severe acute pain in the lumbar area.

She initially attended her general practitioner who diagnosed musculoskeletal pain and she was given a course of physiotherapy, anti-inflammatories (brufen), and told to take a few weeks off work. However, the back pain persisted.

Her general practitioner tried various analgesics, such as paracetamol, co-codamol and co-proxamol with no real effect. She needed numerous episodes off work and became mentally low and frustrated. She was worried that the management would be angry with her and felt she was letting the team down.

The general practitioner became exasperated with Kate's frequent visits and eventually sent her for a magnetic resonance imaging (MRI) scan, which demonstrated a disc bulge at the L3/L4 level of her lumbar spine. She was referred to the orthopaedic surgeons and underwent a surgical decompression. This procedure helped for a short time. However, the pain gradually returned to the same severity and it was Kate's suggestion that she be referred to the local pain clinic.

It was nearly 15 months since her pain first started when she was seen at the clinic by the pain consultant and her pain was obviously chronic. By this time she was on half salary, depressed and very anxious about her future. The consultant took a full history, examined her, assessed her pain and reviewed her current analgesic regime. Kate complained of shooting, stabbing pain radiating through her buttock down her left leg (caused by irritation of the sciatic nerve). She was commenced on gabapentin 300mg three times a day for the neuropathic pain and the dose was gradually titrated up to 600mg three times a day. The consultant also suggested that she try a TENS machine, a course of acupuncture and booked her in for an epidural of steroids and local anaesthetic. This combination of treatments controlled the pain to some extent, but over the following year Kate needed a repeat epidural and 10 sessions of acupuncture. She was then referred to the pain management programme to teach her relaxation techniques and self-management coping strategies to learn to live with the pain.

Kate continues to need regular epidurals and acupuncture and uses her TENS machine. Unfortunately she has had to take early retirement due to her ongoing symptoms.

It is important to remember that there may well be no cure for chronic pain but hopefully symptoms can be ameliorated.

STOP

Now consider your own practice:
- Has your area of work a specific chronic pain team?
- Familiarise yourself with how to contact them.
- Perhaps you could spend time with the team on the wards or in an out-patient setting.
- Do all patients have a baseline pain assessment on admission?
- Does your area of work have pain assessment charts to enhance your assessment?
- Are they being used regularly to reassess the patient's pain?
- Does your area have pre-printed pain care plans?
- Is the pain documentation in use? If not discuss with your mentor.
- Are there any barriers to good pain management?

Implications for nursing practice

■ The under-treatment of chronic pain can have serious outcomes including emotional, social and physical effects.
■ Be aware of your own prejudices, biases and misconceptions.
■ The best treatment for chronic pain is multidisciplinary.
■ Include the patient in the treatment plan.
■ Patients may be reluctant to engage in some treatments for fear of causing themselves more harm.

Key points

■ The principles of chronic non-malignant pain management are:

- Medical assessment of the underlying cause.
- Belief in the patient's report of pain.
- Measurement of the patient's pain.
- Selection of the most appropriate therapy.
- Discussion of the goals of treatment.
- Reassessment as often as needed.

■ Chronic pain is a pain state that is ongoing.
■ The underlying cause of chronic pain cannot be 'cured'.
■ Chronic pain serves no purpose.
■ Chronic pain is under-treated.

References

Breivik H (2003) *New Data to Confirm the Magnitude of Chronic Pain as a Health Problem in Europe*. Pain in Europe Meeting: Prague.

International Association for the Study of Pain (1986) *Classification of Chronic Pain. Descriptions of Chronic Pain*. International Association for the Study of Pain: Seattle.

McCaffery M (1983) *Nursing Management of the Patient in Pain*. JB Lippencott: Philadelphia.

Useful addresses

British Pain Society
21 Portland Place, London W1B 1PY
Tel: 020 7631 8870
Website: www.britishpainsociety.org

Neuropathic Trust
PO Box 26, Nantwich, Cheshire CW5 5FP
Tel: 01270 611 828
Email: info@neurocentre.com
Website: www.neurocentre.com

Pain Concern
PO BOX 13256, Haddington EH41 4YD
Tel: 01620 822 572
Website: www.painconcern.org.uk

Oxford Pain Internet Site
Website: www.jr2.ox.ac.uk

The Pain Web
Website: www.thepainweb.com

CHAPTER 7

Pain in palliative care

Gill Arnold, Jane Lee and Peter Stuart

Introduction

Pain is often the most dominant symptom suffered by cancer and palliative care patients and is frequently the reason why patients initially present to their general practitioner. Health care professionals, patients and their families associate suffering from cancer with suffering from severe, debilitating and constant pain. Incorrect and under-treatment of cancer pain continues to be a major health care problem and can be attributed to, among other things, misconceptions of the prevalence of cancer pain and a fatalistic attitude of health care professionals (Furstenberg *et al*, 1998). Although cancer patients can be found in all areas of health care practice, some nurses may treat very few patients with cancer pain, while for others the problem is more prevalent. This can give the nurse an unbalanced understanding of the prevalence of cancer pain and it is therefore important to have an overall awareness of the incidence of the problem.

In advanced cancer 65–88% of patients will experience pain (Morita *et al*, 1999) (see *Table 7.1*). Several studies have demonstrated that the incidence of pain increases with the progression of disease and that the primary site of the cancer can determine the severity of the pain (Hoskin and Makin, 2003) (*Table 7.2*). In addition the severity of the pain varies depending on the extent of the disease, its progression and the therapeutic interventions (Doyle *et al*, 2004). *Table 7.3* helps to clarify this by classifying the pain associated with the cancer into groups of causes (Hoskin and Makin, 2003). The nurse needs to have a basic understanding of the incidence and causes of cancer pain to be able to assist in the alleviation of patients' suffering.

Why assess pain?

Careful assessment of a patient's pain is vital in order to establish its possible causes, and to promote understanding of the impact it is having on the patient's life (Bennett *et al*, 2005). The initial assessment will provide the basis for evaluating the effectiveness of analgesics and other interventions. Assessment of pain should be an ongoing process in order to ensure that the patient's pain continues to be controlled.

Table 7.1: Symptom prevalence and incidence

	Prevalence on admission(%)	Incidence until death(%)
Anorexia	57	94
Pain	65	88
General malaise	58	77
Constipation	33	71
Fever	26	70
Dyspnoea	33	66
Oedema	27	65
Dry mouth	25	61
Incontinence	23	50
Cough/sputum	29	48
Nausea/vomiting	29	48
Death rattle	6	44
Abdominal swelling	26	42
Pleural effusion	27	32
Somatitis	7	26
Paralysis	23	25
Ascites	27	23
Diarrhoea	7	23
Myoclonus	0	13
Headache	4	9
Itching	3	9

Table 7.2: Site of cancer and severity of pain

Primary site	Severity of pain: Patients surveyed (%)			
	None	Mild	Moderate	Severe
Prostate	17	22	20	41
Oesophagus	29	21	13	38
Gynaecological	10	10	47	33
Colorectal	21	21	27	32
Haematological	13	29	26	32
Head and neck	17	11	43	29
Lung	26	23	30	21
Breast	22	25	31	21
Stomach	26	30	26	17

Table 7.3: Classification of cancer pain by cause

Pain directly caused by cancer (primary and metastatic)	*Pain caused by cancer treatment*
Bone invasion	Surgery
Soft tissue infiltration	Late radiation effects
Nerve pain	Chemotherapy
Visceral pain	

Pain associated with progressing malignant illness	*Incidental pain unrelated to cancer (examples)*
Pressure areas	Osteoarthritis
Infection	Angina
Musculoskeletal	Peripheral vascular disease, etc.
Tension headache	
Colic	
Dyspepsia	

Assessing the patient with pain

The first assessment involves taking a pain history from the patient. Careful attention should be paid to communication, ensuring that the patient is comfortable and understands the aim of the interview. The assessor needs to be aware of any non-verbal cues the patient may give about the pain.

Experience will aid health care professionals to develop their own approach to assessing pain and taking a pain history. The phrasing of the questions is not important, but it is necessary to develop a logical sequence of questions in order to obtain a clear picture of the patient's pain (Watson *et al*, 2005).

The following types of questions may be asked.

- How long have you had the pain?
- Where is the pain?
- Can you describe the pain?
- How severe is the pain?
- Is the pain there all the time?
- What makes the pain worse?
- What makes the pain better?
- Does the pain stop you from doing things?
- Does the pain wake you at night?
- What painkillers have you been taking?
- Have they helped?

Assessment tools

The use of pain assessment tools gives the health care professional a better understanding of patients' pain from their perspective (Bennett *et al*, 2005). Using an assessment tool also ensures that the effectiveness of any interventions can be accurately assessed. However it must be remembered that these tools should be used as part, not the whole, of the assessment process. Patients need to be encouraged to describe their experience of pain in their own way.

There is a wide variety of assessment tools available, such as simple-to-use visual analogue scales, numerical rating scales, verbal rating scales and body charts. These are covered in more detail in *Chapter 3*.

These scales should be completed by patients themselves and not by the health care professional. They provide useful information on the intensity of the pain as experienced by the patient. However because they do not describe the impact the pain has on the patient's life they should only form part of the assessment process.

Pain questionnaires

Pain scales can provide a simple and efficient way of evaluating a patient's pain. However pain is a multidimensional experience and may require a multidimensional assessment tool such as the McGill Pain Questionnaire (Watson *et al*, 2005). Questionnaires should again be completed by the patient, and can be complicated and time-consuming. They are essential as part of the research process and can be helpful when a patient has pain that is difficult to control (Bennet *et al*, 2005).

Types of pain

Cancer pain can be categorised into different types; the type depends upon the organs or body structure involved.

Neuropathic pain

Neuropathic pain is a pain that is transmitted by a damaged nervous system (Watson *et al*, 2005). There are many potential causes for neuropathic pain in cancer and these are outlined in *Table 7.4* (Twycross and Wilcock, 2002). Many patients describe neuropathic pain as a sensation of shooting, radiating, burning or shock-like pain arising from damage in the peripheral or central nervous system.

Visceral pain

Pain that arises from the visceral organs of the body such as the liver, stomach, uterus and thoracic viscera may be caused by pressure and stretching. Patients

Table 7.4: Causes of neuropathic pain in advanced cancer

Cancer	Nerve compression/infiltration
	Spinal cord compression
	Plexopathy
	Thalamic tumour
	Debility
	Post-herpetic neuralgia
Anti-cancer or other treatment	Chronic surgical incision
	Phantom limb pain
	Chemotherapy – peripheral neuropathy
	Radiation fibrosis – plexopathy
Concurrent disorders	Diabetic neuropathy
	Post-stroke pain

may complain of cramping or colicky pain. Visceral pain is sometimes 'referred' and is felt in other parts of the body away from the site of unpleasant stimulation, for example diaphragmatic pain often refers to the shoulder-tip. Visceral pain may be associated with other symptoms such as nausea and vomiting.

Bone pain

Bone pain is often described as severe and can be difficult to treat. It can be constant with an increase in severity on movement or weight bearing depending on where it is. This type of pain can lead to further complications due to reduced movement and mobility, for example, limited rib movement may lead to increased risk of chest infection. If bone metastases are present the best way to manage such pain is with radiotherapy.

Soft tissue pain

Soft tissue pain is often described as a throbbing pain or like a muscle spasm. It arises from damage to the skin and deep tissues and is usually localised.

Pharmacology

The World Health Organization three-step analgesic ladder for cancer pain presents a simple scheme for providing adequate pain relief (Inturissi *et al.*, 1990). Step one is treatment with a non-opioid analgesic, step two is treatment with an opioid analgesic and step three is opioid plus non-opioid analgesics.

Adjuvant drugs can be used at all levels. See *Chapter 2* for a diagrammatic representation of the ladder. The two underlying principles are:

- If the pain is not controlled at one level then a move to the next level is required, not another drug from the same level.
- Continuous pain requires continuous analgesia.

There is no top to the ladder, ie. there is no maximum dose for strong opioids.

Non-opioids

This group includes paracetamol, which is a synthetic, centrally-acting non-opioid (Twycross and Wilcock, 2002) and non-steroidal anti-inflammatory drugs (NSAIDs). NSAIDs are of benefit for pain associated with inflammation, for example, bone pain and soft tissue pain (Twycross and Wilcock, 2002). Commonly used NSAIDs include ibuprofen and diclofenac.

Opioids

Codeine, dihydrocodeine and tramadol should be added to, not substituted for, a non-opioid. If ineffective when given regularly a weak opioid should be changed to a strong opioid, not changed for another weak opioid.

Opioids for moderate to severe pain include morphine, diamorphine, fentanyl, oxycodone, hydromorphone, buprenorphine and methadone (for specialist use only).

Morphine is the strong opioid of choice for moderate to severe cancer pain (Watson *et al*, 2005).

Titration of morphine

Start with immediate release morphine in liquid or tablet form.

- The dosage should be four hourly.
- The same dose should be prescribed 'as required' with no time limit.
- The patient should be encouraged to ask for breakthrough medication.
- A laxative should always be prescribed.
- An anti-emetic may be needed.

Once patients' requirements are steady they can be converted to a controlled release preparation.

- Total the morphine required for the last 24 hours including 'as required' morphine and divide by two for the twice daily dose.

- An 'as required' dose for breakthrough pain should always be prescribed. This is calculated as one sixth of the total daily dose prescribed, with no time limit.

If after 24–48 hours the patient's pain is not controlled, the dose should be increased. The new dose can be calculated as above by adding up the total (regular plus 'as required') oral morphine required over the last 24 hours and dividing by two to give the twice daily controlled-release dose. This will usually result in a dose increase of 30–50%, which is a safe and effective increase (Bennett *et al*, 2005). The 'as required' dose for breakthrough pain should also be increased.

STOP
Further advice may be obtained from the palliative care team.
Does your area have such a team? Do you know how to access it?

Side-effects of strong opioids

Possible side-effects should be discussed with patients when they are started on opioids.

Nausea and vomiting
Nausea occurs in 30–60% and vomiting in 10% of patients commenced on opioids (Bennett *et al*, 2005). It usually settles within a week and can be controlled by a regular anti-emetic such as metoclopramide or cyclizine. If it persists then an alternative opioid should be considered.

Constipation
Ninety-five percent of patients on opioids suffer from constipation (Bennett *et al*, 2005). This is a result of the action of opioids on the gut and the spinal cord which results in reduced intestinal secretions and peristalsis (Inturissi, 1990). This is a long-term problem and all patients taking opioids should also be prescribed a softening and stimulant laxative.

Drowsiness
Mild drowsiness is common when patients first start an opioid and this symptom should wear off after a couple of days (Watson *et al*, 2005). The patient may need explanation and support during this time. If the drowsiness persists or is of an unacceptable level a switch to an alternative opioid should be considered.

Other side-effects of opioids are dry mouth, sweating, itching, hallucinations and myoclonic jerking.

Misconceptions around use of opioids

Both patients and health care professionals may have concerns around the use of strong opioids. These are usually based on fears of addiction and tolerance on the part of the patients while health care professionals tend to worry about respiratory depression and sedation. However, when used correctly and carefully opioids cause few problems (Bennett *et al*, 2005). The possibility that the patient may have concerns about the use of opioids must be borne in mind by the health care professional and opportunity given for discussion.

Addiction
This does not occur when opioids are used for managing pain. If the cause of the pain is removed, for instance by a nerve block, then the opioid can be reduced or stopped with no problems. If the opioid is stopped it should be done gradually as there may be a physical dependence.

Tolerance
Patients are often concerned that there is a need to 'save' strong painkillers for when they are really needed, ie. in advanced disease. This is not the case; tolerance to opioids is extremely rare and because there is no maximum dose the dose can be increased as required.

Breakthrough pain
According to Caraceni *et al* (2004) breakthrough pain is 'a transitory flare of pain that occurs on a background of relatively well-controlled baseline pain'.

This type of pain is also referred to as episodic and incident pain. The term incident pain may be used more specifically to describe pain related to movement. If incident pain is a problem, precipitating factors should if possible be identified and avoided or 'as required' analgesia given.

If the patient is experiencing pain regularly before the next dose of analgesia is due, the regular dose may need to be increased.

Opioid rotation

This term is used to describe the change from one strong opioid to another, eg. from morphine to oxycodone. This is done because the patient develops uncontrolled adverse effects such as severe sedation, confusion or nausea and vomiting on the current dose of opioid (Mercadante, 1999). Changing the patient to an alternative strong opioid often produces an improvement in pain control, frequently with a lower dose and with a reduction in side-effects. Changing to an alternative opioid requires an understanding of the conversion ratios.

Case study: Opioid rotation

Mrs M, a 79-year-old woman with ovarian carcinoma, has low pelvic pain which responds to morphine. However she is very sleepy on her current dose of 20mg MST twice daily. She is switched to oxycodone 10mg twice daily with 5mg oxynorm as required which provides good pain control and complete resolution of her drowsiness.

Specialist analgesics

There are a number of drugs used by specialist palliative care practitioners that have not been included in the above. These drugs can have significant side-effects or require careful use because of their toxicity and contra-indications which is why they are not more widely used. These drugs tend only to be used in hospices or specialist settings, but you may come into contact with patients on such drugs in your area and so an awareness of their use is important. See *Table 7.5* for a list of commonly used specialist analgesics (Twycross *et al*, 1998). Before making any changes to these medications it is advisable to discuss the changes with the patient and with the specialist palliative care team. If you are in any doubt about their use in individual patients or need further support and advice it is advisable to contact the specialist palliative care team for your area.

Adjuvant analgesics

The primary action of adjuvant drugs is often not pain relief, but they may have been found to produce analgesia as a secondary effect. They can be used in combination with drugs on all steps of the WHO analgesic ladder.

Adjuvant analgesics include:

- antidepressants, eg. amitripyline
- anticonvulsants, eg. gabapentin, carbamazepine
- corticosteriods, eg. dexamethasone
- antispasmodics, eg. buscopan
- muscle relaxants, eg. baclofen, diazepam
- bisphosphonates, eg. pamidronate, zoledronic acid
- N-methyl-D-aspartate acid (NMDA) receptor channel blockers, eg. methadone, ketamine.

Antidepressants and anticonvulsants may be useful for neuropathic pain, which does not always respond to the combined use of a strong opioids and an NSAID. Corticosteroids are helpful for pain and weakness associated with nerve root/nerve trunk compression and spinal cord compression, and they also

Table 7.5: Specialist analgesics used in cancer pain management

Drug	Indication/dosage/side-effects
Methadone	
Indication	Intolerable adverse effects with morphine, morphine hyperexcitability, poor pain response to morphine, pain relief needed in severe renal failure
Dosage	Half life of 8–75hr that can be longer in older patients
Side-effects	As with morphine but made more difficult to manage due to long half life. Is protein binding and accumulates in tissues when given repeatedly, creating a reservoir of methadone making accumulation a problem
Ketamine	
Indication	Neuropathic, inflammatory and ischaemic pain unresponsive to standard therapies
Dosage	Starting dose and route vary. SC 10–25mg prn. CSCI starting dose 0.1–0.5mg/kg/hr, increasing by 50–100mg/24hr; maximum reported dose 2.4g/24hr. Orally 25mg qds and prn increasing in steps of 10–25mg
Side-effects	Most patients experience vivid 'ketamine' dreams. Hallucinations can usually be controlled by diazepam, midazolam or haloperidol. 40% of patients complain of hypertension, tachycardia, dysphoria, nightmares, delirium, and nystagmus. Can be very irritable to the skin at injection site
Ketorolac	
Indication	NSAID in injectable form. Severe pain associated with soft tissue and bone metastases poorly responsive to maximum doses of other NSAIDs combined with a strong opioid
Dosage	Can be given by intermittent injections 20–30mg SC tds. Starting dose 60mg/24hr. CSCI. Increase by 15mg/24hr
Side-effects	As with any NSAID inhibits platelet aggregation so should be used with caution in patients with peptic ulceration, gastrointestinal bleeding, cerebrovascular bleeding or asthma. Should also be used with caution in hepatic impairment, furosemide, ACE inhibitors, methotrexate and lithium

SC, subcutaneous; CSCI, continuous subcutaneous infusion, NSAID, non-steroidal ani-inflammatory drug; ACE, angiotensin converting enzyme reduce oedema associated with inflammatory conditions and tumour growth. Antispasmodics are used for patients with visceral distension pain and colic, for example, in intestinal obstruction. Relaxing the smooth muscle can relieve this spasm. Muscle relaxants are used for painful muscle spasms (cramp). Bisphosphonates are osteoclast inhibitors and are used to relieve metastatic bone pain. Lastly, NMDA receptor channel blockers such as ketamine and methadone are used primarily for neuropathic pain when standard analgesics are ineffective.

Barriers to effective pain relief

Despite widely available published guidelines for effective pain management, most notably the World Health Organization analgesic ladder (1986) (See *Chapter 2*), 45% of patients in early stages of cancer and 75% of patients in advanced stages experience at least some pain (Goudes *et al*, 2001).

An abundance of literature suggests that barriers to adequate pain relief are influenced by a number of factors including health care professionals, patients, and in certain cases the patient's family or carers. Health care professionals do not always have standardised education and clinical experience. This can lead to shortcomings in their knowledge with regard to opioid pain relief, including issues surrounding addiction, tolerance and side-effects (Agency for Health Care Policy and Research, 1994).

Patients may hamper their own treatment due to similar misconceptions about the use of opioids. They can also be reluctant to report pain for a variety of reasons including: belief that the pain is inevitable or untreatable, fear that the disease is getting worse, and concerns about not being a 'good' patient and bothering the nurses and doctors.

Total pain

The concept of total pain is now well established in the hospice and palliative care setting, however its existence is often debated outside of these areas and consequently often overlooked and misunderstood (Furstenberg *et al*, 1998). Patients complaining of total pain may have no biomedical explanation for the severity of the pain leading to health care professionals questioning its validity. Total pain refers to pain that is not only physical but also social, spiritual and psychological and was initially described by Cicely Saunders in the 1960s to describe pain that includes the entire illness including mental and spiritual suffering and using descriptions of pain such as 'desolation', 'bitterness', 'meaninglessness', and 'abandonment' (Strang, 2004).

Total pain is complex and subjective but describes the impact that physical pain has on other dimensions of an individual. It encompasses the patient's mood, attitude, life experience, resources, coping mechanisms and family response (Greenstreet, 2001). In the context of cancer pain it is a continual reminder of the presence of the cancer and, as the pain becomes worse, an indication to the patient of the progression of the disease, which can dominate daily life (Hoskin and Makin, 2003). Zaza and Baine (2002) identify an association between cancer pain and different coping styles.

Managing total pain can be challenging but also rewarding for the nurse. Nurses have reported feelings of inadequacy and helplessness when caring for patients with uncontrolled pain (Arber, 2004). It is too easy to make the assumption that the pain is not real but in the patient's mind, however the nurse should take seriously the patient's complaint of pain and the patient's distress should be recognised and understood (Faull and Woof, 2002). The role of the nurse in managing total pain is to acknowledge, with the patient, that the pain is real and can encompasses all aspects of the patient's life beyond physical sensations. Additionally the nurse needs to develop a sympathetic and supportive relationship with the patient that allows the patient to feel heard and understood. The nurse, with the assistance of the wider multidisciplinary team, needs to employ non-medical strategies that facilitate more positive coping mechanisms to address and resolve all aspects of total pain. They need the support of their peers to allow the time to offer a truly holistic approach to patients and their families (Greenstreet, 2001; Arber, 2004).

Case study: Total pain

Mr Brown is a 64-year-old patient with advanced bladder cancer. His cancer has now metastasised to the liver with locally advanced disease. He also has significant co-morbidity of heart disease, obesity and early arthritis, as well as a history of depression.

On assessment he has pain in his lower back, pelvis, thighs, abdomen and left thorax. A recent skeletal survey shows degenerative diseases in the spine but no metastases. He is currently prescribed MST 80mg bd, oramorph 20mg prn, diclofenac 50mg tds, and co-codamol 8/500 qds.

Mr Brown reports no benefit from MST and oramorph and therefore does not take it as prescribed. He feels the co-codamol provides the most effective analgesia. His family is very concerned about his pain and become quite anxious when he reports feeling uncomfortable.

An assessment of Mr Brown's pain scored his back pain as a constant 2/10 in severity. The pain is described as a toothache in the back. The thigh, abdominal and thorax pain appear to be resolved, although Mr Brown is vague about this. Previously his pain had been very severe, prior to starting MST, keeping him awake at night and preventing him from mobilising. It was at this time that the urologist told him the cancer had advanced and would not benefit from surgery. His heart disease prevents him being given chemotherapy.

It was identified that there was a psychological component to Mr Brown's pain. When patients are experiencing 'total pain', analgesia alone may not resolve the symptoms. Allowing Mr Brown the time to discuss his fears and anxieties may help to manage his pain.

Mr Brown perceived no benefit from using oramorph and therefore was reluctant to use it. This may be because the dose was too small for the severity of the pain, or it was the wrong drug. By encouraging Mr Brown to take it more, and offering support, the effect and dose of the opiate can be monitored more closely.

Good supportive care, allowing Mr Brown the time to talk about his worries and anxieties, as well as an increase in opiate dose significantly helped to improve his pain management.

Impact of pain on the family

It is not unusual for a patient's family to be involved with care and, as a result, the family caregiver often takes on the burden of the patient's pain. The consequence of unrelieved pain for the family caregiver may include tension, depression, anxiety, sleep disturbance, impaired health and poor nutritional status, as well as disruptions to family relationships and financial burden (Yates *et al*, 2004). Emotionally, caregivers report overwhelming feelings of grief, burden, frustration, and helplessness when their loved ones experience pain (Redinbaugh *et al*, 2002). The result is that the treatment of cancer pain goes beyond the pain experienced by the patient and should be extended to the patient's family.

It is difficult to shield family carers from the emotional burden of caring. They often take on the role of surrogate advocate for the patient, describing their role as 'pain managers' who make decisions about the patient's analgesia and when he or she should or should not receive it (Redinbaugh *et al*, 2002). It must be remembered that this role is often undertaken out of love and care for the patient with a genuine belief that what the carer is doing is right for the patient. However this can lead to conflict with nursing staff when the carer's perceptions about the patient's pain and method of management are considered, by the nurse, as inappropriate. In addition Redinbaugh *et al* (2002) found that family carers who reported greater levels of distress regarding their loved one's pain were less accurate in estimating the patient's level of pain tending to over-estimate the severity, which could lead to increased conflict with nursing staff.

The role of the nurse in addressing the impact pain can have on the family is to recognise the positive benefits family caregivers can have on the patient's pain. Caregiver misconceptions often arise from a lack of knowledge and understanding of the causes of cancer pain and its appropriate management. It is not unusual for carers to seek information from many sources including other family members, leaflets and the Internet. The disadvantage with some of these sources is that the information may be inaccurate or inappropriate leading to further misconceptions, eg. about the use of opiates.

Poor communication has been shown to be a contributory factor in inadequate pain management (Yates *et al*, 2002). However carers are often keen to work with health care professionals to address pain (Yates *et al*, 2004). The nurse should recognise this and utilise the opportunity to address any anxieties due to misunderstandings by providing relevant and accurate information and helping the carer find positive ways of managing the patient's pain. Techniques such as massage and distractional therapies can be helpful.

Pain at the end of life

Pain is one of the most common and feared symptoms experienced by patients at the end of life. However, pain continues to be under-treated, largely due to the barriers previously discussed.

As patients become weaker they find it increasingly difficult to take oral medication. Therefore non-essential drugs should be stopped and drugs that need to continue may have to be given via an alternative route. Pain management at end of life may rely heavily on opioid analgesics, from moderate opioids such as codeine and dihyrocodeine to strong opioids such as morphine.

The subcutaneous route is generally recommended when oral medication is no longer an option, either bolus doses, or if regular doses are required, a continuous subcutaneous infusion should be commenced. This method has the advantage of maintaining constant levels of the drug and avoids the potential stress of the use of multiple needles.

When choosing an opioid analgesic consideration of delivery and dose options, potential side-effects, efficacy of the agent, duration of action and patient's age need to be taken into account to ensure maximum benefit with minimal side-effects.

Throughout the terminal phase it is important to continue treatment with opioid analgesia even when the patient is sedated or unresponsive as if an opioid is stopped abruptly the patient may experience withdrawal (Inturrisi, 2002).

Ethical considerations

The World Health Organization (2004) recognises the increasing complexity of the ethical issues in the care of patients with progressive and serious illness. The practice of nursing involves many ethical responsibilities of which advocacy, accountability, co-operation and caring are some of the concepts that provide a foundation for the nurses' ethical decision making (Fry and Johnstone, 2002). The ethical issues are too extensive to give an in-depth analysis of the application of such principles in the management of cancer pain in this chapter. The aim is to provide a basic awareness of some of the issues the nurse should be concerned about when addressing pain in cancer patients.

To summarise, the main ethical principles applied to health care are: autonomy, beneficence, non-maleficence, justice, veracity and fidelity (Beauchamp and Childress, 2001). How these principles are applied will differ, depending on situation and cultural context, but they are generally regarded as the core framework for ethical decision making in health care (Fry and Johnstone, 2002). In addition to these principles, the Nursing and Midwifery Council's (NMC) *Code of Professional Conduct* (2004) and the International Council of Nurses' *International Code of Ethics for Nurses* (2000) dictates the moral and ethical behaviour of the nurse. For example, in the context of pain, the *International Code of Ethics for Nurses* requires the nurse to alleviate suffering, for which pain is clearly a cause. The NMC *Code of Professional Conduct* dictates that nurses have a duty of care to the patient to provide safe competent care and nurses are personally accountable for their own practice and answerable for their own actions and omissions. To apply this principle to the management of a patient's cancer pain the nurse is accountable for administering or omitting analgesia and having appropriate knowledge of the analgesia prescribed. During periods of uncontrolled pain the patient's dignity and interests can be compromised. In such instances the NMC (2004) requires the nurse to identify the patient's preferences regarding care and holds the nurse accountable for promoting and respecting the patient's interests and dignity.

A more specific ethical issue regarding analgesia is based on the doctrine of double effect. This is a complex idea based on the principle that a single act may have two foreseen effects or intentions, one good and one harmful. The first intention should be to do good and the bad effect foreseen but not intended (Beauchamp and Childress, 2001). The doctrine of double effect has been extensively debated and more in-depth analysis of the principle can be easily accessed as can any of the ethical points raised. While there is plenty of literature available to increase nurses' awareness of ethical thinking, in reality the problems nurses may face could be more complex and difficult to address. Under such circumstances nurses should seek the support and guidance of their peers and members of the multi-disciplinary team, or, in extreme circumstances, the NMC.

Implications for nursing practice

- Nurses need to have a basic understanding of the incidence and causes of cancer pain to be able to assist in its relief.
- Assessment of pain should be an ongoing process in order to ensure that the patient's pain continues to be controlled.
- The principles of the WHO ladder should be followed when considering analgesic options.
- Side-effects should be discussed with patients prior to the commencement of opiates.
- Nurses need to recognise the positive benefits family and caregivers can have on a patient's pain and support them in this role.

Key points

- Pain is often the most dominant symptom in cancer and palliative care patients.
- Careful assessment of a patient's pain is vital in order to establish its possible causes and to promote understanding of the impact it is having on the patient's life.
- Nurses, patients and carers may hamper effective treatment due to misconceptions about analgesic medication.
- Pain is one of the most common and feared symptoms experienced by patients at the end of life.
- When oral medication is no longer an option other delivery methods need to be implemented quickly.

References

Agency for Health Care Policy and Research (1994) Management of cancer pain. Patient guide. *Oncology Nurses Forum* **21**: 1232–8.

Arber A (2004) Is pain what the patient says it is? Interpreting an account of pain. *Int J Palliat Nurs* **10**(10): 491–6.

Beauchamp T, Childress J (2001) *Principles of Biomedical Ethics* (5th edn.) Oxford University Press: New York.

Bennett M, Forbes K, Faull C (2005) The principles of pain management. In C Faull, Y Carter, R Woof (Eds.) *Handbook of Palliative Care* (2nd edn.) Blackwell Publishing: Oxford.

Caraceni A, Martini C, Zecca E (2004) Breakthrough pain characteristics and syndromes in patients with cancer pain. An international survey. *Palliat Med* **18**: 177–83.

Doyle D, Hanks G, Cherny N, Calman K (2004) *Oxford Textbook of Palliative Medicine* (3rd edn.) Oxford University Press: Oxford and London.

Faull C, Woof R (2002) *Palliative Care: An Oxford Core Text*. Oxford University Press: Oxford.

Furstenberg C,. Ahles T,. Whedon M, Pierce K, Dolan M, Roberts L, Silberfarb P (1998) Knowledge and attitudes of health-care providers toward cancer pain management: A comparison of physicians, nurses, and pharmacists in the State of New Hampshire. *J Pain Sympt Manag* **15** (6): 335.

Fry S, Johnstone M (2002) *Ethics in Nursing Practice* (2nd edn.) Blackwell Publishing: Oxford.

Goudes L, Carr D, Bloch R, Balk E (2001) *Management of Cancer Pain*. Evidence Report No 35. AHRQ Publication.

Greenstreet W (2001) The concept of total pain: A focused patient care study. *Brit J Nurs* **10**(19): 1248–55.

Hoskin P, Makin W (2003) *Oncology for Palliative Medicine* (2nd edn.) Oxford University Press: New York.

Inturrisi C (2002) Clinical pharmacology of opiates. *Clin J Pain* **18**: 3–13.

International Council of Nurses (2000) *The ICN Code of Ethics For Nurses*. International Council of Nurses: Geneva, Switzerland.

Mercadante S (1999) Opioid rotation for cancer pain. *Cancer* **86**(9): 1856–66.

Morita T, Tsunoda J, Inoue S, Chihara S (1999) Contributing factors to physical symptoms in terminally-ill cancer patients. *J Pain Sympt Manag* **18**: 5.

Nursing and Midwifery Council (2004) *The NMC Code of Conduct: Standards for Conduct, Performance and Ethics*. Nursing and Midwifery Council: London.

Redinbaugh E, Baum A, DeMoss C, Fello M, Arnold R (2002) Factors Associated with the Accuracy of Family Caregiver Estimates of Patient Pain. *J Pain Sympt Manag* **23**: 1.

Strang P, Strang S, Hultborn R, Arner S (2004) Existential pain – An entity, a provocation, or a challenge? *J Pain Sympt Manag* **27**(3): 241–50.

Twycross R, Wilcock A (2002) *Symptom Management in Advanced Cancer*. Radcliffe Medical Press: Oxford.

Twycross R, Wilcock A, Thorp S (1998) *Palliative Care Formulary*. Radcliffe Medical Press: Oxford.

Watson M, Lucas C, Hoy A, Back I (2005) *Oxford Handbook of Palliative Care*. Oxford University Press: Oxford.

World Health Organization (2004) *Palliative Care: The Solid Facts*. WHO Regional Office for Europe: Copenhagen, Denmark.

Yates P, Aranda S, Edwards H, Nash R, Skerman H, McCarthy A. (2004) Family caregivers' experiences and involvement with cancer pain management. *J Palliat Care* **20**(4): 287.

Yates P, Edwards H, Nash R, Walsh A, Fentiman B, Skerman H, McDowell J, Najman J (2002) Barriers to effective cancer pain management: A survey of hospitalized cancer patients in Australia. *J Pain Sympt Manag* **23**(5): 393.

Zaza C, Baine N (2002) Cancer pain and psychological factors: A critical review of the literature. *J Pain Sympt Manag* **24**(5): 526–42.

World Health Organization (2986) *Cancer Pain Relief*. World Health Organization: Geneva.

CHAPTER 8

The management of pain in children

Sarah Roberts

Introduction

The International Association for the Study of Pain (1979) defines pain as, 'An unpleasant sensory and emotional experience with actual or potential tissue damage or described in terms of such damage.' It goes on to say, 'Pain is always subjective; each individual learns the application of the word through experiences related to injury in early life.' This definition recognises the importance of pain experiences in childhood and the effects they have on an individual throughout life. However there is a wealth of evidence to suggest that children's pain is often under-assessed and under-treated (Schechter *et al*, 1991; Bernstein *et al*, 1991). The reasons for this are many and varied; children's communication about pain may be misinterpreted; children's behavioural responses may differ from adults; and children and babies may not be given adequate analgesia due to the fears health care professionals have about using opioids in this group.

Although the belief that children do not feel as much pain as adults has been disproved there are still a great many inconsistencies in the assessment and treatment of children's pain.

Assessment of pain in children

The first stage in managing pain in babies and children is obtaining a thorough and accurate assessment. This is not as straightforward as it sounds as children's ages, cognitive ability, behaviour, culture and communication skills will vary greatly, for example, it is no use asking 2-year-olds to rate the severity of their pain using a 0–10 scale as they have not yet developed that degree of numerical thinking. Children will sometimes find it difficult to localise their pain or they may use words that an adult might not immediately recognise as related to pain, for example, a 6-year-old boy who had undergone a below knee amputation described his stump as 'beaming', which to him meant intense pain. Children may have had only limited experiences of pain prior to coming into contact with health care professionals and therefore relate all pain to an experience they remember, an example of which is the young child who describes 'a headache in my tummy'.

The Royal College of Nursing report *Ouch! Sort It Out* (1999a) contains many children's descriptions of pain which were gained using interviews, play scenarios, stories, drama and picture drawing. One child said, 'Pain squashes you, it is as if your bones are being pushed in', another described pain by saying, 'It's all spiky inside' and a third stated, 'It felt like a tickle rather than a pain, not a nice pain but a sharp pain tickle.' These three examples illustrate the many and varied ways children describe pain. It is vital therefore that nurses are aware of this and strive to fully understand the child by further questioning and observation.

STOP

Think about words or phrases you used to describe pain when you were a child or those you have heard children using. Are they instantly recognisable as meaning pain?

With a group of colleagues each write down the words you use to describe pain then ask each other how you would interpret them if a child in your care used them.

In order to gain some consistency and allow children's pain to be recorded numerous pain assessment tools have been developed for use by health care professionals. Twenty two of these tools were evaluated in the Royal College of Nursing (1999b) clinical practice guideline *The Recognition and Assessment of Acute Pain in Children*. Scales have been developed to assess pain in children and babies from the ages of 0 to 18 and range from a simple choice of a number to more detailed assessments involving several pages of questions. At the University Hospitals of Leicester three assessment tools have been combined to enable all ages of children to have their pain assessed and documented in a consistent way (*Figure 8.1*). The FLACC tool (Merkel *et al*, 1997) is a behavioural rating scale that allows the nurse to assess a baby or young child's pain using five categories:

- facial expression
- leg movement
- activity
- crying
- consolability.

The Faces tool is an adaptation of scales described by various authors (Bieri *et al*, 1990; McGrath *et al*, 1985; Whaley and Wong, 1987) and

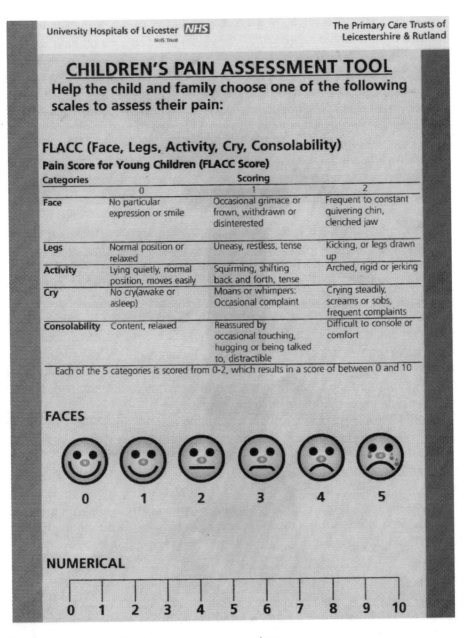

Figure 8.1: An example of a pain assessment chart.

comprises six cartoon faces in various stages of pain (ranging from none to severe). This type of tool is described as a self-report scale and is generally considered suitable for children over the age of 4 years. The child is encouraged to choose the face that best describes their level of pain. The advantage of this tool is that it allows children to self-report their pain and it is quick and easy to use. The disadvantages are that children may choose the face that relates to how happy they are rather than how much pain they are in and they may choose the face they like best. It is therefore important that a thorough explanation is given to the child and family. Relating the faces to pain the child has already suffered may be helpful, e.g. asking 'What face was your pain when you grazed your knee, had a tummy ache, bumped your head, etc.' Doing this allows children to make better use of the tool if they suffer pain in hospital. This is easily achieved when a child is in hospital for an elective procedure where there is time to prepare but much more difficult when a child is admitted to hospital already suffering pain. In this case the child should receive appropriate analgesia as a matter of priority before the tool is explained.

The numerical scale is a self-report scale commonly used with adults and has been found to be useful when assessing pain in older children and adolescents. As with the Faces tool a thorough explanation is essential to allow the child/young person to make best use of it. As with all self-report scales children may either under- or over-score their pain depending on what they perceive the consequences to be. For example, if a child knows their discharge may be delayed if they report pain they may under-score themselves; conversely if a child's parents buy gifts and treats when they are in pain they may score themselves higher. It is however of vital importance not to challenge a child's self-report but to use it in addition to behavioural signs to plan an individual pain-relief regime.

In order for a pain assessment scale to be useful it needs to be reliable and easy to use for both children and health professionals. As mentioned previously there are a great many tools available and different institutions will use different ones. The important thing is that some type of validated tool is being used and that the child's scores are documented and acted on. Pain scoring should be given as high a priority and carried out with the same frequency as observations of temperature, pulse and respirations although often this is not the case.

STOP

What tool, if any, does your institution use?

Is it used consistently and are scores acted on? If not why do you think that is?

As well as using pain assessment tools nurses need to be vigilant in observing for emotional and behavioural signs of pain in children and babies. Assessment tools for babies and young children rely heavily on these signs and consideration should also be given to these signs when caring for older children and young people. Just because a child is not crying or verbalising pain does not mean that they are pain free.

Behavioural signs of pain may include:

- changed behaviour (in order to assess this you will need to ask parents or carers how the child is normally)
- irritability
- screaming/crying/sobbing/whimpering
- aggressiveness
- unusual quietness
- disturbed sleep pattern
- lethargy
- restlessness
- loss of appetite
- reluctance to move
- unusual posture
- refusal to move
- lying 'scared stiff'.

Physiological signs of pain can be observed in children and babies that are similar to those that adults display and are described in more detail in the pervious chapters on adult pain assessment. However when caring for children and babies in areas outside of the intensive care environment behavioural indicators and self-report should always be the mainstay of pain assessment.

Parents should always be involved in pain assessment with children although it has been shown that they may under- or over-estimate their child's pain (Bellman and Paley, 1993). This could be for a variety of reasons; the parents' own pain experiences, their parenting style, the nature of the child's injury or illness (for example, if parents and children are facing a life-threatening illness pain may be rated higher), etc. Parents need support and clear explanations from health care professionals in order to assist in their child's pain assessment and management.

STOP

Obtain copies of some of the pain assessment tools available for children and babies. Read the descriptions below then answer the questions:

What pain assessment tool would you use with each child and why?
Rate the children in order of priority providing a rationale for your choice.

- *Ella, age 2, has been admitted with pneumonia. Every time she coughs she cries and holds her head. She is clingy with her parents. She has had a dose of paracetamol 2 hours ago.*

- *George, aged 4 months, has just returned from theatre following a hernia repair. He is crying loudly. On further inquiry you learn that he has had some analgesia in theatre. His mum is very anxious and demanding loudly that something is done.*
- *Hannah, aged 11, has been admitted with a broken arm. She is lying quietly on her bed holding her arm and appears uninterested in her surroundings. She has not had any analgesia since she arrived on the ward 4 hours ago. Her parents have gone home.*
- *Rosie, aged 8, had several teeth extracted one day ago. She is refusing to eat and screams loudly if the nurses try to do anything for her. Her mum is beginning to get cross with her as she cannot be discharged until she has eaten.*
- *Gareth, aged 11, had orthopaedic surgery to both legs 2 days ago. On questioning he says he is fine but is often seen to be grimacing if he tries to move in bed and the night staff report that he has had a disturbed night's sleep.*

Did you find the exercise easy to complete?
Do your colleagues agree with your rating?

There are no right or wrong answers to this exercise, however, it should illustrate to you that pain assessment in children should involve the consideration of many factors and your findings should be used to plan care.

The QUESTT approach to pain assessment in children as described by Wong and Baker (1988) provides a useful and easily remembered summary to assist the health care professional when caring for children in pain.

QUESTT stands for:

- Question the child.
- Use pain rating scales.
- Evaluate behavioural and physiological changes.
- Secure the parents' involvement.
- Take the cause of pain into account.
- Take action and evaluate the results.

Management of pain in children

As with adults pain management techniques in children can be separated into two main categories: pharmacological and non-pharmacological techniques. The most successful pain management plan usually involves a combination of both.

Pharmacological methods

For information on appropriate doses of analgesic drugs refer to the current edition of the *British National Formulary* for children.

For information on the mode of action of the following drugs please refer to *Chapter 2*.

Paracetamol

The most common analgesic drug used with children and babies is paracetamol. It is readily available to parents and health care professionals and comes in a variety of preparations which enables it to be given to the majority of children. Paracetamol is most commonly given orally in the form of either a suspension or tablet and doses can be easily calculated as appropriate to the child's age and weight. Paracetamol suppositories are available, however, their absorption is slower than the oral preparations and often a larger dose needs to be given. Recently an intravenous preparation of paracetamol has become available which allows the drug to be given to children who are nil by mouth and either cannot or will not have suppositories. Paracetamol is a safe drug if given in appropriate doses, however it is very dangerous in overdose and therefore it is of the utmost importance to educate parents/carers in an appropriate dosing regime prior to discharging children home.

Non-steroidal anti-inflammatory drugs (NSAIDs)

NSAIDs are also used commonly in children in pain; examples of these are ibuprofen, diclofenac and naproxen. They may be given orally or rectally. Only one type of NSAID should be given at any one time. These drugs are useful in a variety of situations including post-operatively, in children with broken bones and/or soft tissue injuries and in children with rheumatological conditions. These drugs should not be given to children with clotting abnormalities or where there is a significant risk of bleeding as they may interfere with platelet function. They should be used with caution in children with asthma as they may cause bronchospasm.

Opioid analgesics

Opioid analgesics such as codeine (classed as a weak opioid) and morphine (classed as a strong opioid) are frequently given to children in hospital particularly post-operatively or in children suffering with oncological conditions. Opioid analgesics can be given alongside paracetamol and an NSAID, as all have different modes of action, to provide what is known as multi-modal analgesia. Codeine is available as an oral solution or tablet and often causes constipation so children should be prescribed a stimulant laxative if they are on regular doses. Morphine can be given orally (as a solution or tablet), rectally, subcutaneously, intramuscularly (although this is not advocated in conscious children), intravenously and via an epidural.

Children, their parents and some health care professionals may worry about children becoming addicted to opioid analgesics. In reality this is rarely a problem when these drugs are used in appropriate doses to relieve pain. It is the job of the nurse to reassure parents and children of that and ensure that the child receives appropriate doses and monitoring when these drugs are used. Information leaflets detailing the actions of analgesic drugs can be helpful in reinforcing any verbal advice given. If parents/carers still have anxieties then it may be appropriate to involve the pharmacist and/or anaesthetist in helping to educate them about the risks and benefits of these drugs.

Analgesic drugs should be given regularly to children and babies in order to prevent pain. Nurses should be aware that children will suffer pain as a result of illness, surgery or injury and therefore nurses should not wait for children to be in severe pain before administering 'as required' medication. Giving regular multi-modal analgesia achieves the most balanced pain relief for children as it maintains fairly constant blood levels of the drugs. If a child is not given regular analgesia pain will increase and with it anxiety and it will be difficult to gain control of the child's pain quickly. In hospital it is worth discussing with parents and children if they would like to be woken for analgesia at night as this may avoid them going long periods without medication and consequently waking in pain.

One way of ensuring that children receive appropriate levels of analgesia is to use continuous intravenous infusions of drugs, the most common being morphine. Older children (usually above 6–7 years) can achieve high quality pain control by using patient controlled analgesia (PCA) similar to that used by adults but on a regime worked out according to their weight. The use of epidural analgesia is gaining popularity as a method of post-operative pain relief in babies and children as it can provide high quality analgesia. Children and babies on continuous infusion, PCA or epidural analgesia should still be given drugs from the other analgesic groups to obtain the best possible levels of pain control

For more information on PCA and epidurals please see *Chapter 2*.

Non-pharmacological methods

There are many non-pharmacological methods of pain relief suitable for use by and with children. These include:

- aromatherapy/massage
- relaxation
- guided imagery
- play therapy
- transcutaneous nerve stimulation (TENS).

Health professionals should aim to support all the physical and emotional needs of both the child and the family when treating pain. Non-pharmacological methods are relatively cheap and easy to use and can be taught to parents and children for use at home. Most hospitals do not have policies and guidelines for therapies such as aromatherapy and massage due to the lack of a broad evidence base and therefore nurses are unable to use them. However the benefits of relaxation are widely known and relaxation therapy can be used very successfully with children in pain.

Relaxation

All children subjected to pain whatever the cause will suffer some anxiety, fear and sadness related to their experience. It has been shown that there is a positive relationship between anxiety levels and pain perception (Brugal, 1971). Pain or the anticipation of pain is seen as a threat by most humans and threat causes activation of the sympathetic nervous system. This causes the physical changes known as the 'fight or flight response', characterised by an increase in heart rate, blood pressure, respiratory rate, acuity of the senses, blood flow to voluntary muscles, blood glucose and sweat gland activity (Payne, 2000). Relaxation can help to calm this response by increasing the activity of the parasympathetic nervous system which reverses these changes (Benson, 1976). The reduction in muscle tension can have great benefits to the child in pain as holding muscles tense can in itself produce pain, leading to a vicious circle of pain, anxiety and muscle tension.

Relaxation methods suitable for use with children can be simple and easy to learn. Using bubbles and the analogy of 'blowing the pain away' can help children to relax by controlling their breathing. Asking children to imagine that they are a rag doll and gradually relaxing areas of the body can also be very useful.

STOP

What do you find relaxing? Could you use this to help if you were in pain? What methods do you think children and young people would find useful?

Guided imagery

This technique involves the child being guided through an image of their choice by a facilitator who asks questions such as, 'What can you see? What can you smell? How does it feel?', etc. The facilitator's questions are guided by the child's response. This has been described as 'engaging the child's imagination and concentration on a specific event to modify a particular response' (Doody *et al*, 1991). This technique can be used to provide distraction and pain relief for children undergoing procedures as well as those suffering more lasting pain. Children should be encouraged to choose an image in which they would like to participate and in which they feel in control. Once the image is chosen the child is encouraged to relax by whatever method works for the individual. This may take practice and some trial and error. Facilitators should engage children and attempt to win their trust for the imagery to be successful. This technique requires training and practice and should not be undertaken by an inexperienced practitioner. It is however a very useful technique to learn in order to help children in pain.

Play therapy
Children will use play as a distraction technique when they are in pain. They can be assisted in this by hospital play specialists who are experts in using play as a means of distraction. If a play specialist is not available then it is the nurse's duty to provide and facilitate play activities with children in pain.

Transcutaneous nerve stimulation
This technique can be used in children in pain. Please see *Chapter 6* for an explanation of its use.

Special circumstances

Neonates

Neonates include infants up to 28 days old. Until relatively recently it was believed that very young babies did not feel pain. However, there is now much evidence to disprove this (Anand and Hicky, 1987; Fitzgerald *et al*, 1989). How much pain neonates feel is impossible to tell but anyone who has assisted in taking blood from babies will realise that the baby feels pain. Indeed it has been shown that even unborn babies feel pain when a needle is inserted.

How would you know a baby was is pain rather than hungry?
There are various tools available to assist in the assessment of pain in this group some of which are evaluated in the Royal College of Nursing (1999) guideline, *The Recognition and Assessment of Acute Pain in Children*. Most assess a mixture of behavioural signs, facial expression, crying and physiological signs. A study of neonates undergoing painful procedures noted withdrawal movements, squirming, cardiovascular and respiratory changes, facial expression and crying (Craig *et al*, 1993).

One example of an assessment tool is CRIES (Krechel and Bildner, 1995) (*Table 8.1*) which is used to assess post-operative pain in neonates. The infant is assessed using the five parameters and the scores added together to get a final score of between 0 and 10 in a similar way to the FLACC tool. It is quick and easy to use but has the disadvantage that recording blood pressure may upset the infant and also oxygen saturations may be lowered for reasons other than pain.

Table 8.1: The CRIES assessment tool

Parameter	Score 0	Score 1	Score 2
Crying	None	High pitched	Inconsolable
Requires oxygen to keep oxygen saturations above 95%	No	Less than 30% oxygen	More than 30% oxygen
Increased vital signs	Heart rate and blood pressure equal to or below pre-operative values	Heart rate and blood pressure increased less than 20% over preoperative values	Heart rate and blood pressure increased more than 20% over preoperative values
Expression	None	Grimace	Grimace/grunt
Sleepless	No	Wakes at frequent intervals	Constantly awake

The treatment of pain in neonates is still hampered by fears of giving opioids to this group because it is known that they metabolise these drugs comparatively slowly. It has been found that during medical and nursing education the hazards of using opioids are reinforced while appropriate therapeutic use of these drugs is rarely discussed (Yaster and Deshpande, 1988). There are however no reasons why infants in pain should not receive adequate analgesia and the *British National Formulary* for children has comprehensive information on appropriate dosing regimes.

Adolescents

The psychological changes taking place in adolescence can cause a huge amount of emotional turmoil and when pain is added young people may find it hard to express how they are feeling and how to deal with their pain. Most adolescents trust health care professionals to assess and treat their pain adequately, however it has been shown that nurses often rate pain lower than adolescents (Hilliard and Le Baron, 1982). Nurses are often unsure how to react to an adolescent in pain and whereas they may instinctively provide physical comfort in the form of cuddles to a younger child they may feel this is inappropriate for an adolescent. It is important to find a way for young people to express their pain and the use of a simple 0–10 scale is often useful. Giving young people responsibility in the assessment and management of their pain allows them to feel in control of the situation. The use of PCA is particularly helpful in this group as long as frequent assessments of pain are made and reassurances given that the young person cannot overdose.

Helping young people to express chronic pain

Children may suffer from chronic pain as a result of a variety of medical conditions, such as sickle cell disease, juvenile arthritis, cancer or degenerative disorders or it may be of unknown causes. The treatment and assessment of this type of pain differs from that of acute pain in that the pain has no foreseeable end. As a result children may suffer from emotional and psychological problems which in turn impact on their ability to express and cope with pain. Assessment will focus on the nature, site, severity and frequency of the pain, what coping strategies the child uses and an assessment of the anxiety the pain causes. Pain diaries are useful for helping children express in their own words how the pain makes them feel and also how it impacts on their life. Children can be encouraged to express their pain by drawing or writing stories and, in some cases, using media such as drama can be very beneficial. It is also important to involve parents in the assessment process and address their anxieties alongside those of their child.

STOP

Imagine you are a parent of a child who is suffering chronic pain as a result of juvenile arthritis.

How do you think you would feel, what words would you use to describe your feelings?

The treatment of chronic pain in children needs a team approach with input from professionals of many disciplines including:

- nursing
- medical
- psychology
- physiotherapy
- occupational therapy
- pharmacy
- play specialists
- teaching.

A clear management plan should be formulated which must be reviewed regularly and adjusted according to the child's condition. The child and family must be involved in formulating the management plan as it is something they will have to live with day to day. Children and their parents need to be helped to minimise the effect that pain has on their lives and learn coping strategies in order to do this.

Conclusion

It must be remembered that babies and children suffer pain in the same way that adults do. The expression of pain will depend on a variety of factors including age and cognitive ability. It is the nurse's responsibility, when caring for the child in pain, to make a thorough assessment using appropriate tools and to document the findings.

Following detailed and accurate assessment, action must be taken to relieve the pain appropriately using pharmacological and non-pharmacological methods. Regular evaluation will measure the effectiveness of interventions and allow for rapid treatment changes.

Parents should be involved in all aspects of their child's pain management and given clear explanation of all treatments. Parents will need support from the nurse in order to be able to help their child.

The nurse caring for the child in pain should acknowledge the distress pain causes and strive to minimise this at all times.

Implications for nursing practice

- Children express pain in a different way to adults.
- Despite an immature nervous system neonates do feel pain.
- Children may not always be truthful about their pain but nurses must never say they disbelieve their self-report.
- It is possible to assess pain in all ages of children using validated assessment tools.
- Parents should be involved in their child's pain assessment.
- Pain in children can be treated with pharmacological and non-pharmacological approaches.

Key points

■ Children's pain is often under-assessed and under-treated. It is the responsibility of the nurse to ensure that a thorough assessment using appropriate tools is undertaken and evaluated regularly.

■ Adolescents may have difficulty expressing their pain. Nurses are often unsure how to react to the adolescent in pain.

■ Children with chronic pain need to be helped to minimise the effect that pain has on their lives and learn coping strategies in order to do this.

■ Analgesia should be given to children on a regular basis and not as required.

■ Parents need support and clear explanation from health care professionals in order to assist in their child's pain assessment and management.

References

Anand KJS, Hicky PR (1987) Pain and its effects in the human neonate and fetus. *New Engl J Med* **317**: 1321–9.

Bellman MH, Paley CE (1993) Pain control in children. Parents underestimate children's pain. *Brit Med J* **307**: 1563.

Benson H (1976) *The Relaxation Response*. Collins: London.

Bernstein B, Schechter NL, Hickman T (1991) Pre-medication for painful procedures in children: Aa national survey. *J Pain Sympt Manag* **6**: 190.

Bieri D, Reeve RA, Champion GD, Addicoat L, Ziegler JB (1990) The Faces Pain Scale for the self-assessment of the severity of pain experienced by children: Development initial validation and preliminary investigation for ratio scale properties. *Pain* **41**: 139–50.

Brugal MA (1971) Relationships of pre-operative anxiety and post-operative pain. *Nurs Res* **20**(1): 26–31.

Craig KD, Whitfield MF, Grunau RVE, *et al* (1993) Pain in the preterm neonate: Behavioural and physiological indices. *Pain* **52**: 287–99.

Doody SB, Smith C, Webb J (1991) Non-pharmalogical intervention for pain management. *Crit Care Nurs. Clin N Amer* **3**(1): 69–75.

Fitzgerald M, Millard C, McIntosh N (1989) Cutaneous hypersensitivity following peripheral tissue damage in newborn infants and its reversal with topical anaesthesia. *Pain* **39**: 31–6.

Hilliard JR, Le Baron S (1982) Relief of anxiety and pain in children and adolescents with cancer: Quantitative measures and clinical observations. *Int J Clin Exp Hypnosis* **30**(40): 417–42.

International Association for the Study of Pain (1979) Cited in Carter B (Ed.) (1994) *Child and Infant Pain: Principles of Nursing Care*. Chapman and Hall: London.

Krechel SW, Bildner J (1995) CRIES: A new neonatal postoperative pain measurement score.

Initial testing of validity and reliability. *Paediatr Anaes* **5**: 53–65.

McGrath PA, Develoer LL, Hearn MJ (1985) Multidimensional pain assessment in children. *Adv Pain Res Ther* **9**: 387–93.

Merkel S, Voepel-Lewis T, Shayevevitz JR, Malviya S (1997) The FLACC: A behavioural scale for scoring postoperative pain in young children. *Pediatr Nurs* **23**(3): 293–7.

Payne R (2000) Relaxation Techniques. *A Practical Handbook for the Health Care Professional*. Churchill Livingstone: Edinburgh.

Royal College of Nursing Institute (1999a) *Clinical Practice Guidelines: Ouch Sort It Out: Children's Experiences of Pain*. Royal College of Nursing: London.

Royal College of Nursing Institute (1999b) *Clinical Practice Guidelines:The Recognition and Assessment of Acute Pain in Children*. Royal College of Nursing: London.

Schechter NL, Bernstein B, Beck A, Hart L, Scherzer L (1991) Individual differences in children's responses to pain: Role of temperament and parental characteristics. *Paediatrics* **87**: 171–7.

Whaley L, Wong DL (1987) *Nursing Care of Infants and Children*. Mosby: St Louis, MO.

Wong DL, Baker CM (1988) Pain in children: Comparison of assessment scales. *Pediatr Nurs* **14**: 9–17.

Yaster M, Deshpande JK (1988) Management of paediatric pain with opioid analgesics. *J Paediatr* **113**(3): 421–9.

CHAPTER 9

Physiotherapy in the management of chronic pain

Paul J Watson

Physiotherapy is well established in both acute and chronic pain. A physiotherapy referral is the most commonly used pathway for patients with musculoskeletal pain. Indeed referral to physiotherapy if an acute episode of pain fails to improve with routine analgesia is part of national guidelines for the management of low back pain and whiplash associated disorder (Waddell and Burton, 2001; Staal *et al*, 2003, Wadell, 2004).

Critics have suggested that evidence for the effectiveness of physiotherapy has been lacking and that the research has suffered from poor methodology resulting in ambiguity. Not all of this criticism is fair; physiotherapy is rarely offered clinically as a single modality. Physiotherapists see the musculoskeletal system as a whole and correcting local dysfunctions such as restricted joint motion is often only part of the process. Exercise, physical activity retraining and education are all essential components of rehabilitation. To separate treatments into the component parts and, for example, compare the effectiveness of exercise with manipulation in the restoration of movement would, in the mind of the physiotherapist, set up a clinical nonsense in the name of research. Having said this the supporting evidence for the use of physiotherapy in the management of chronic pain is presented.

The full range of electrotherapies is not covered in this chapter, rather the important role physiotherapy has in regaining function and rehabilitation is the focus. This does not mean the issue of treating pain is ignored. There is very good evidence that exercise and the restoration of normal function is particularly effective in reducing the report of pain.

Manual therapies

Manual therapy refers to hands on therapies of massage, soft tissue mobilisation/manipulation and the more familiar mobilisation/manipulation of joints. Massage has fallen out of favour with physiotherapists, partly because of the physiotherapy profession's perception of the negative image it conveys about it but also because of the lack of evidence for the effectiveness of the treatment. The fact that this therapy is also time-consuming to perform properly might also have led to its restricted use. Recently, massage has received a boost to its reputation following a review of the evidence that suggested it can be effective in treating low back pain (Furlan *et al*, 2002). Massage follows a number of different forms but the treatments of interest here are traditional massage and acupuncture-like massage. Traditional, often called Swedish, massage appears to be less effective than massage which focuses on local tender or trigger points, ie. acupuncture massage. The evidence however is less clear when one examines the research; the best outcomes from massage are seen when it is combined with advice and exercise (Furlan *et al,* 2002).

In acute and sub-acute conditions where inflammation is present massage can be effective in reducing swelling and removing oedema (De Domenico and Wood, 1997). Massage can also stimulate blood flow through tissues and perform very localised stretches (De Domenico and Wood, 1997). However in chronic pain conditions there is little evidence of substantial ongoing inflammation and swelling and compromised blood flow has only been described in certain myofascial pain syndromes. This begs the question of how massage might be effective in the management of pain. The possible reasons why massage might have an effect have surprisingly been given little attention despite its widespread use in the management of pain. The effects of massage are likely to be as a result of stimulation of Aβ receptors and the relaxation effect of the treatment itself (Clay and Pounds, 2002). Reductions in muscle activity and self-reported reduction in perceived stress and anxiety are common findings immediately following massage (Hernandez-Reif *et al*, 2001). Intriguing research has demonstrated neurohormonal changes including increased levels of serotonin and reduced levels of cortisol (Hernandez-Reif *et al*, 2005), both of which have a modulatory effect on pain.

It has been suggested that acupuncture-like massage reduces pain by stimulating the endogenous opioid system (Hernandez-Reif *et al*, 2005). The treatment certainly focuses on tender points and acupuncture points in the same way as acupuncture but there is no clear evidence that there is an opioid response.

STOP

Have you ever used massage to help a painful condition? Did it help?
Have you ever rubbed a pain better ?

Soft tissue mobilisation

Soft tissue mobilisation is where the therapist manually moves and stretches tissues to regain extensibility. This is often combined with other massage techniques. Such techniques are used to mobilise and break down adhesions within and between tissues which may limit movement and normal performance

(De Domenico and Wood, 1997). Deep friction is a specific type of very localised and forceful mobilisation over underlying bone which aims to break localised adhesions and develop a localised inflammation in chronic conditions (Brosseau *et al*, 2003).

Joint mobilisation and manipulation

These therapies are commonly used to treat spinal pain and movement dysfunction. They are probably the most commonly performed therapies used by the musculoskeletal physiotherapist. They are rarely applied as a stand alone treatment and normally are performed as a part of treatment that will include education and exercise (Grieve, 1994; Haldeman and Hooper, 1999).

Joint mobilisation refers to movement of the joint within the available range of motion. This might be beyond the range patients can themselves achieve during movement. Manipulation is a small amplitude high velocity thrust action at the end of the range of motion taking the joint beyond the available range of motion and the reader will be familiar with this as an osteopathic type of manipulation often accompanied by an audible crack (Grieve, 1994; Halderman and Hooper, 1999; Broome, 2000). Increased range of motion immediately following manipulation is well documented and there is little doubt that manipulation performs this very useful service, in the short-term at least (Broome, 2000). Proponents of manipulation argue that restoring range of motion speeds up the recovery process, restores the normal joint biomechanics, reduces pain and helps in the prevention of further injury or recurrence of pain (Broome, 2000). Joint mobilisation increases range of motion through repeated stretching and deformation of the tissues which increases the extensibility of joint structures. Reinstatement of the normal range of motion and biomechanical integrity has been the main treatment effect for both mobilisation and manipulation.

Biomechanical responses to manipulation and mobilisation are not the only explanatory mechanisms by which treatments might be effective. Manual therapy involves stimulation of a wide variety of tissues and the physiological effect of this has only recently received attention. Activation of a manipulation-induced analgesia has been suggested and data from a number of studies have demonstrated an increase in pain thresholds following manipulation and this has been used to explain the reduction in pain that has been observed following such procedures (Cote *et al*, 1994; Wright, 1995). Descending inhibition via the peri-aqueductal grey matter has been suggested as a putative mechanism.

Manual therapies have been criticised as being 'passive' where the patient is the recipient of treatment rather than being actively involved in it and learning to self-manage the condition. The importance of self-management is emphasised in the management of chronic pain problems because the epidemiology tells us that chronic and recurrent pain are by their nature ongoing problems which, although manageable with judicious use of interventions, cannot be 'cured'. For this reason it is essential that patient are taught strategies for self-management. Over the years physiotherapists have been exhorted to take a biopsychosocial approach to chronic pain and adopt some of the lessons learned from the pain management approach developed in multidisciplinary pain management programmes. Although some practitioners still feel more comfortable with a biomedical approach to pain a wider perspective is becoming more accepted.

Exercise

Exercise is one of the cornerstones of physiotherapy and it serves a number of functions. Chronic pain and the limitations it inevitably imposes on the individual have a number of long-term consequences. At its worst very disabled patients will experience physical deconditioning (Bortz, 1984) whereby the activity limitation leads to a number of adverse physiological changes.

It is an undisputed fact that pain limits physical activity but it must be remembered that, in modern society, few people are really physically active and so widespread general deconditioning only occurs in those who suffer the greatest limitation. Most people with a chronic pain problem continue with their regular routine of work and housework, which for many people is the only regular physical activity they take. However, more specific problems occur because people avoid certain activities that aggravate their pain and so, although widespread deconditioning is not common in many people with chronic pain (Wittink *et al*, 2000), local weakness or limitation of movement is. Patients seen in physiotherapy outpatient departments are unlikely to be grossly physically deconditioned but people seen on pain management programmes are much more likely to display the so called 'deconditioning syndrome', the features of which include (Bortz, 1984):

- Muscle weakness.
- Limited muscle endurance.
- Loss of flexibility of soft tissues and joints leading to restricted range of motion.
- Loss of cardiovascular function and endurance.
- Loss of movement accuracy and impaired co-ordination.
- Loss of lean body mass and increase in adiposity.

There is much research to demonstrate that specific exercises have specific physiological effects. Repeated low load exercise tends to improve endurance whereas high load low repetition exercise increases strength. However, rehabilitation in its true form is not simply a series of exercises to correct a dysfunction. Rehabilitation requires a more integrated approach to treatment.

An integrated biopsychosocial approach to physiotherapy

As stated earlier, physiotherapy should not be seen as a single modality; few therapists operate solely as manual therapists or exercise therapists. Manual and exercise therapy are very specific treatments that can be useful in addressing specific dysfunctions. However, the patient needs to be able to translate improvements made in these treatments into improvements in physical performance and valued activities of daily living. The broader objectives of a physiotherapy pain management approach are as follows (adapted from Watson, 2003):

- Assist patients in altering their belief that their problems are unmanageable and beyond their control.
- Inform patients about their condition.
- Assist patients to move from a passive to an active role in the management of their condition through engagement in physical activity.
- Help patients to monitor reasons for not engaging in activity and identify how these are influenced by internal and external events.
- Give patients a feeling of competence in the execution of positive strategies in the management of their condition.
- Help patients to develop a positive attitude to exercise and personal health management.
- Help patients to develop a programme of paced activity to reduce the effects of physical de-conditioning.
- Assist patients to develop an activity programme that can be developed once contact with the clinician has ended.

The remainder of this chapter examines the elements that enable these treatment goals to be achieved.

Goal setting and pacing

Chronic pain patients often report levels of activity that fluctuate dramatically over time. On questioning at initial assessment, they report that they frequently persist in activities until they are prevented from carrying on by the pain experienced. This leads them to rest until the pain subsides or until frustration moves them to action whereupon they then try again until defeated by the increase in pain.

In the acute and subacute stage avoidance of normal activity can lead to problems. Guidelines for the management of painful conditions recommend a return to usual activity as soon as possible. Most people manage this with little support but continued avoidance can lead to disability, and returning to strenuous activity too early can result in prolonged healing or risk of re-injury.

Gil and colleagues (1988) described pacing as moderate activity–rest cycling. It is a strategy that enables patients to control exacerbations in pain by learning to regulate activity and, once a regime of paced activity is established, to gradually increase their activity level. The converse of this is the 'overactivity–pain–rest' cycle (Gil *et al*, 1988) where the patient rests but then becomes frustrated and returns to usual activity too quickly, the result of which may be re-injury and/or exacerbation of pain.

The purpose of goal setting is to regulate daily activities and to structure an increase in activity through gradual pacing-up. Activity is paced by time or by the introduction of quotas of exercise interspersed by periods of rest or a change in activity (Keefe *et al*, 1996; Johansson *et al*, 1998; Marhold *et al*, 2001). The advice to 'rest' or 'take it easy' is often given to a patient in the acute stage but what constitutes rest is rarely explained and how to return to usual activity in a structured way is not addressed – both are required.

Goals are set in three separate domains: physical, which relates to the exercise programme patients follow and which sets the number of exercises to be performed or the duration of the exercise and the level of difficulty; functional/task, which relates to the achievement of functional tasks of everyday living such as housework or hobbies; and social, in which patients are encouraged to set goals relating to the performance of activities in the wider social environment (Watson, 2000). It is important that goals are specific, measurable, achievable, personally relevant and have a time frame. Patients will always pursue highly valued goals even in the face of increased symptoms (Affleck *et al*, 2001) so it is important that the patient values the goals. Continued goal-attainment will reinforce the patient's perception that they are in control (Bandura, 1994). It is therefore important that goals are set which encourage success but are sufficiently challenging to assure progress. The setting of short-, long-term and immediate goals should be a matter of negotiation between patients and their therapists.

Physical exercise

Limited physical capacity in chronic pain is due to a myriad of factors (Watson, 1999). Tight scar tissue or shortened soft tissues may limit movement so that certain activities become difficult and the patient starts to avoid them. Altered muscle tension, posture and muscle activity in response to an original injury may persist and be reinforced by psychological factors and habit (Main and Watson, 1996). Treatment must address obvious problems such as weakness or dysfunction, but a generalised exercise programme is suitable for most patients with chronic pain (Watson, 2000).

Exercise in the management of pain can be divided into three components,

- stretching
- strengthening
- cardiovascular (aerobic) conditioning.

There is no compelling evidence to date that specific exercise has any benefit over general exercise in the management of musculoskeletal pain, but the consensus of opinion is that aerobic exercise and the promotion of an active lifestyle is beneficial (Faas, 1996; Waddell and Burton, 2004). This does not mean that specific exercises should not be undertaken where an obvious problem exists (eg. obvious unilateral weakness of a painful limb) but it is only part of an activity plan. Concentrating on specific exercises should not divert the clinician from getting the patient back to normal everyday function.

Stretching and range of motion exercises

Pain may have started with an initial injury or pathology, or started insidiously. Although the pain may be widespread there may be areas where the effects are felt most. Stretching exercises need to be general and comprehensive to address the general loss of flexibility, as well as specific to the individual's needs.

Motion only through a restricted range results in limitation of joint range through the shortening of joint soft tissue structures and an impoverishment of joint nutrition. Motion through complete joint range is required to assist in the nutrition of the cartilage of synovial joints as well as in the maintenance of the length and strength of the joint capsule, ligaments and muscles.

Stretches should be static/sustained where the muscle is taken to its limit and the stretch is maintained for at least 5–6 seconds, although many authors suggest longer. Bouncing or ballistic stretching should not be used. Combining muscle relaxation or a simple warm up regime with stretching will increase the effectiveness of the stretch.

Stretching should form part of the patient's daily routine especially in warm up and warm down sessions. Goal setting will encompass increases in the length of time the stretch is maintained as well as the number of stretches performed. Patients report that introducing regular stretching into daily work and home routines, especially between different activities and after periods of static work (eg. reading, typing) is extremely helpful.

Strengthening

Loss of muscle strength and endurance has been identified in many types of chronic pain. Exercises aimed at increasing the strength and endurance of muscle groups is an established component of physiotherapy treatments. Furthermore increased physical activity improves neuromuscular co-ordination. Monitoring an increase in strength in particular can be motivating for some patients, although the increases are most often attributed to improvement in the patient's confidence in performing the activity rather than to physical strength alone (Watson, 2000).

Like most physical training modalities there are many differing ideas on what is the best way to increase muscle strength. A general rule of thumb is that strength training occurs when the muscles are exercised at an intensity of greater than 40% of maximal force with a relatively low number of repetitions; any lower force than this and a higher number of repetitions would tend to increase endurance. Exercise at greater intensity than this tends to increase muscle bulk and strength. Very high percentages of maximal force (greater than 60%) with low repetitions give the greatest increases in maximal force as an effect of training (Olsen and Svendsen, 1992). It is unlikely that people with chronic pain conditions will be able to participate in such intensive exercise so intensities of 40% are more realistic. However, some patients may find even this level of intensity difficult in the early stages of rehabilitation.

Aerobic conditioning

Aerobic exercise should be presented within the goal setting and pacing approaches and patients should be given information on how it relates to a healthy lifestyle as well as to pain management. Aerobic conditioning has demonstrated improvements in pain distribution, depression, and physical capacity (Burkhardt *et al*, 1994; Wigers and Stiles, 1996; Haldorsen *et al*, 1998; Brosse *et al*, 2002). The relationship between improvements in physical capacity/fitness and reductions in self-reported disability is mixed. Some have found no association between physical improvement and reduced disability (Jensen *et al*, 1994; Hildebrandt *et al*, 1997). Where an association is found it has only explained a small amount of the variance for improvement (Burns *et al*, 1998; Mannion *et al*, 2001). The contribution of improvements in physical function is often overshadowed by the importance of changes of psychosocial factors.

Paced walking, swimming, stationary exercise cycling, stair walking, use of a stair climber and non-impact aerobic classes have all been suggested as ways of increasing physical fitness (Watson, 2000). The exercises should be performed at least three times each week for best effect. Where possible patients should exercise to 60–70% of aerobic capacity or should pace themselves up to achieve this level of intensity if maximum improvement in cardiovascular function is to be gained. However, the relationship between the intensity of the exercise and the improvement in disability is unclear and even less intense programmes can be effective in reducing disability and distress and in improving symptoms

(Mannerkorpi, 2005). It is essential that the exercise can also be continued at home. Paced walking and stair walking are obvious examples that can be continued without special facilities.

Practising feared movements

It seems logical that the way to improve or return to an activity is to do that activity and practise until the required performance is achieved. Many 'rehabilitation' approaches do not seem to have understood this, have forgotten it, or have been seduced by new 'fix-all' exercise prescriptions. It seems a vague hope that improved function can be brought about by sole adherence to a series of abstract exercises. Highly specific exercises that are remote from the activities the patient needs to do in daily life are likely to be less effective than specific management. There is very good evidence that people who fear activities will increase their pain or suffer further injury by avoiding these and similar activities. Waddell *et al* (1993) even went so far as to suggest that it is the fear of pain that is more disabling that the pain itself.

In a series of single case experiments Vlaeyen *et al* (2001) demonstrated that a graded exposure technique where subjects repeatedly practise feared movements can be successful in improving the outcome of treatment over and above the effects of graded non-specific exercise. Subjects were required to identify and grade exercises they were worried about or that they feared would increase their pain or cause damage. These exercises were then practised starting with the least feared and progressing to the most feared. Feedback on performance was given with positive reinforcement to challenge fears. Other researchers have demonstrated that a reduction in fear avoidance is an important determinant of a reduction in disability (Woby *et al*, 2004). However, it is not clear if reducing fear of one specific activity generalises to other feared activities (Crombez *et al*, 2002), neither has research demonstrated that patients will adhere to or become adept at practising feared movements without close supervision. Despite these concerns it would appear logical to include the identification and performance of feared movements in rehabilitation.

Exercise adherence

There is a reduction in exercise adherence following completion of an exercise programme (Lewthwaite, 1990; Proschaska and Marcus, 1994). Wigers and Stiles (1996) found that 73% of patients failed to continue an exercise programme when followed up although 83% felt they would have been better if they had continued.

Continuing with exercise is more likely if the individual finds it interesting and rewarding. Exercising in a gym may not be suitable for all. Some people may not have access to such facilities; others may not be motivated by this form of exercise. Developing activities that are patient and family orientated, and can be integrated into the normal daily routine, will help to improve adherence. Exercise should be part of life not an intrusion into it. Encouraging patients to investigate local swimming or walking groups is one way to foster social links and may lead to improved exercise adherence after contact has finished.

STOP

Have any of your patients complained that physiotherapy has made them worse? Would you advise them to continue or stop the treatment?

Physiotherapy-led cognitive-behaviour therapy

Disability due to pain is not simply dependent on the intensity of the pain or the physical limitation of an injury (Main and Spanswick, 2000). The person's reaction to the condition, his or her beliefs about the cause of the pain and the eventual outcome are key to success or failure in treatment. The efficacy of exercise and increasing activity in managing disability related to pain has been demonstrated. However, psychological factors are key predictors of poor outcome from such treatment approaches. There have been a number of attempts to train physiotherapists to address these issues. Physiotherapists have been trained to deliver exercise orientated programmes within a cognitive-behavioural framework. These have been demonstrated to be better than usual treatment by general practitioners (Frost *et al*, 1998; Klaber Moffett *et al*, 1999) and in one study there was evidence that those who underwent a cognitive-behavioural therapy approach rather than a manual therapy intervention were less likely to consult for back pain in a one year follow up (Hay *et al,* 2005). Although these results are encouraging it remains to be determined what are the required clinician competencies and programme elements to ensure success.

Conclusion

Referral to physiotherapy is one of the commonest treatment routes for the person with a painful condition. There is good evidence for the use of many physiotherapy treatments in the management of pain when compared with treatment as usual (general practitioner treatment) or no treatment. To date current knowledge suggests general aerobic exercise is most effective for chronic pain conditions but specific exercises may be included where there are demonstrable local dysfunctions or problems. Addressing fear of movement is recommended in those who are fearful about re-engaging in everyday activities. Continued participation in an active lifestyle is essential for sustained improvement especially for those with a chronic pain condition.

Implications for nursing practice

- Physiotherapy is an important part of the rehabilitation process, nurses can help patients to manage their pain more effectively by reminding them to perform their physiotherapy exercises regularly.
- Nurses are in a prime position to help patients to develop a positive attitude to exercise and personal health management.
- Continued participation in an active lifestyle is essential for sustained improvement in the patient with chronic pain.
- Be aware of your limitations and recognise the importance of the multidisciplinary team in the management of pain.

Key points

- A physiotherapy referral is often the most commonly used pathway for patients with musculoskeletal pain.
- Exercise, physical activity, retraining and education are all seen as components of rehabilitation.
- Restoring the normal joint biomechanics reduces pain and helps in the prevention of further injury or recurrence of pain.
- Specific problems occur because people avoid certain activities which aggravate their pain.
- Physiotherapy should not be seen as a single treatment modality.

References

Affleck G, Tennen H, Zautra A, Urrows S, Abeles M, Karoly P (2001) Women's pursuit of personal goals in daily life with fibromyalgia: A value-expectancy analysis. *J Consult Clin Psychol* **69**(4): 587–96.

Bandura A (1994) *Self efficacy. Encyclopadia of Human Behavior*. Academic Press: New York: 71–8.

Bortz W (1984) The disuse syndrome. *Western J Med* **141**: 691–4.

Broome R (2000) *Chiropractic Joint Technique*. Boston: Butterworth Heinemann.

Brosse AL, Sheets ES, Lett HS, Blumenthal JA (2002) Exercise and the treatment of clinical depression in adults: Recent findings and future directions. *Sports Med* **32**(12): 741–60.

Brosseau L, Casimiro L, Milne S (2003) Deep transverse friction massage for treating tendinitis (Cochrane review) *Cochrane Library Issue 4*. John Wiley and Sons: Chichester.

Burkhardt C, Mannerkorpi K, Hedenberg L, Bjelle A (1994) A randomised controlled trial of education and physical training for women with Fibromyalgia. *J Rheumatol* **21**: 714–20.

Burns J, Johnson B, Mahoney N, Devine J, Pawl R (1998) Cognitive and physical capacity process variables predict long term outcome after treatment of chronic pain. *J Consult Clin*

Psychol **66**: 434–9.

Clay J, Pounds D (2002) *Basic Clinical Massage Therapy: Integrating Anatomy and Treatment.* Lippincott Williams and Wilkins: Philadelphia.

Cote P, Mior S, Vernon H (1994) The short term effect of a spinal manipulation on pressure pain threshold in patients with chronic mechanical low back pain. *J Manip Physiological Therapeutics* **17**: 364–8.

Crombez G, Eccleston C, Vlaeyen JW, Vansteenwegen D, Lysens R, Eelen P (2002) Exposure to physical movements in low back pain patients: Restricted effects of generalization. *Health Psychol* **21**(6): 573–8.

De Domenico G, Wood EC. (1997) *Beards Massage.* WB Saunders: New York.

Faas A (1996) Exercises: Which ones are worth trying, for which patients, and when? *Spine* **21**(24): 2874–8.

Frost H, Lamb SE, Klaber Moffett JA, Fairbank JC, Moser JS (1998) A fitness programme for patients with chronic low back pain: Two-year follow-up of a randomised controlled trial. *Pain* **75**(2-3): 273–9.

Furlan AD, Brosseau L, Imamura M, Irvin E (2002) Massage for low-back pain: A systematic review within the framework of the Cochrane collaboration back review group. *Spine* **27**(17): 1896–910.

Gil K, Ross S, Keefe F (1988) Behavioural treatment of chronic pain: Four pain management protocols. In: France R, Krishnan K (Eds.). *Chronic Pain.* American Psychiatric Press: Washington: 317–413.

Grieve G (1994) *Modern Manual Therapy of the Vertebral Column.* Churchill Livingstone: Edinburgh.

Haldeman S, Hooper P (1999) Mobilisation, manipulation, massage and exercise for the relief of musculoskeletal pain. In: Wall P, Melzack R, (Eds.) *Textbook of Pain* (4th Edn.) Churchill Livingstone: Edinburgh.

Haldorsen EH, Kronholm K, Skouen JS, Ursin H (1998) Multimodal cognitive behavioural treatment of patients sicklisted for musculoskeletal pain: A randomised controlled study. *Scand J Rheumatol* **27**: 16–25.

Hay EM, Mullis R, Lewis M, Vohora K, Main CJ, Watson P, *et al* (2005) Comparison of physical treatments versus a brief pain-management programme for back pain in primary care: A randomised clinical trial in physiotherapy practice. *Lancet* **366**: 2024–30..

Hernandez-Reif M, Field T, Krasnegor J, Theakston H (2001) Lower back pain is reduced and range of motion increased after massage therapy. *Int J Neurosci* **106**(3–4): 131–45.

Hildebrandt J, Pfingsten M, Saur P, Jansen J (1997) Prediction of success from a multidisciplinary treatment program for chronic low back pain. *Spine* **22**(9): 990–1001.

Jensen MP, Turner J, Romano J (1994) Correlates of improvement in multidisciplinary treatment of chronic pain. *J Consult Clin Psychol* **59**:172–9.

Johansson C, Dahl J, Jannert M, Melin L, Andersson G (1998) Effects of a cognitive-behavioral pain-management program. *Behav Res Ther* **36**(10): 915–30.

Keefe FJ, Kashikar-Zuck S, Opiteck J, Hage E, Dalrymple L, Blumenthal JA (1996) Pain in arthritis and musculoskeletal disorders: The role of coping skills training and exercise interventions. *J Orthop Sports Phys Ther* **24**(4): 279–90.

Klaber Moffett J, Torgerson D, Bell-Sayer S (1999) Exercise for low back pain: Clinical preferences, costs and preferences. *Brit Med J* **319**: 279–83.

Lewthwaite R (1990) Motivational considerations in physical therapy. *Phys Ther* **70**: 808–19.

Main C, Spanswick C (2000) Pain Management: An interdisciplinary approach. Churchill-Livinstone: Edinburgh.

Main CJ, Watson PJ (1996) What harm--pain behavior? Psychological and physical factors in the development of chronicity. *Bull Hosp Joint Dis* **55**(4): 210–2.

Mannerkorpi K (2005) Exercise in fibromyalgia. *Curr Opin Rheumatol* **17**(2): 190–4.

Mannion AF, Junge A, Taimela S, Muntener M, Lorenzo K, Dvorak J (2001) Active therapy for chronic low back pain: Part 3. Factors influencing self-rated disability and its change following therapy. *Spine* **26**(8): 920–9.

Marhold C, Linton SJ, Melin L (2001) A cognitive-behavioral return-to-work program: Effects on pain patients with a history of long-term versus short-term sick leave. *Pain* **91**(1–2): 155–63.

Olsen J, Svendsen B (1992) Medical exercise therapy: An adjunct to orthopaedic manual therapy. *Orthopaedic Pract* **4**: 7–11.

Proschaska J, Marcus B (1994) The transtheoretical model: Application to exercise. In: Dishman R (Ed.) *Advances in Exercise Adherence*. Human Kinetics: New York: 161–80.

Staal JB, Hlobil H, van Tulder MW, Waddell G, Burton AK, Koes BW, *et al* (2003) Occupational health guidelines for the management of low back pain: An international comparison. *Occupational and Environ Med* **60**(9): 618–26.

Vlaeyen JW, de Jong J, Geilen M, Heuts PH, van Breukelen G (2001) Graded exposure in vivo in the treatment of pain-related fear: A replicated single-case experimental design in four patients with chronic low back pain. *Behav Res Ther* **39**(2): 151–66.

Waddell G (2004) *The Back Pain Revolution*. Churchill Livingstone: Edinburgh.

Waddell G, Burton AK (2001) Occupational health guidelines for the management of low back pain at work: Evidence review. *Occupational Med* **51**(2): 124–35.

Waddell G, Burton KA (2004) *Concepts of Rehabilitation for the Management of Common Health Problems*. The Stationary Office: Norwich.

Waddell G, Newton M, Henderson I, Somerville D, Main CJ (1993) A Fear-Avoidance Beliefs Questionnaire (FABQ) and the role of fear-avoidance beliefs in chronic low back pain and disability. *Pain* **52**(2): 157–68.

Watson P (2003) Interdisciplinary pain management in fibromyalgia. In: Chaitow L (Ed.) *Fibromyalgia Syndrome: A Practitioners Guide*. Churchill Livingstone: Edinburgh:129–48.

Watson PJ (2000) The pain management programme: Physical activities programme content. In: Main CJ, Spanswick CC (Eds.) *Pain Management: An interdisciplinary Approach*. Churchill Livingstone: Edinburgh: 285–301.

Watson PJ (1999) Non-physiological determinant of physical performance in musculoskeletal pain. In: Max M (Ed.) *Pain 1999 – An Updated Review*. IASP Press: Seattle, WA: 153–8.

Wigers SH, Stiles T, Pa V (1996) Effects of aerobic exercise versus stress management in fibromyalgia: A 4.5 year prospetive study. *Scand J Rheumatol* **25**: 77–86.

Wittink H, Hoskins Michel T, Wagner A, Sukiennik A, Rogers W (2000) Deconditioning in patients with chronic low back pain: Fact or fiction? *Spine* **25**(17): 2221–8.

Woby SR, Watson PJ, Roach NK, Urmston M (2004) Are changes in fear-avoidance beliefs, catastrophizing, and appraisals of control, predictive of changes in chronic low back pain and disability? *Eur J Pain* **8**(3): 201–10.

Wright A (1995) Hypoalgesia post-manipulative therapy. *Manual Ther* **1**: 11–16.

CHAPTER 10

Psychological aspects of chronic pain treatment

Kate Martin and Laura Ambrose

The aim of this chapter is to give an overview of how psychology contributes towards understanding people with chronic pain and to suggest some interventions to empower them to help themselves. The effects of chronic pain can be all-consuming, pervading many aspects of a person's life. Becoming aware of how we perceive situations and exploring techniques for changing this perception can be useful in helping with these aspects of people's lives as well as their direct experience of pain intensity. Interventions can be used solely or in conjunction with other forms of pain management to help further improvement. This chapter focuses on key factors that research suggests contribute to the experience and effective management of chronic pain. However, it is important to remember that pain is an individual experience, and we can never completely enter into another person's experiences; it is therefore important to acknowledge and treat 'individual' experience as the exclusive entity that it is.

Biopsychosocial model of pain

Traditional models propose that pain is directly linked to and moderated by levels of physical damage; treatment was therefore to identify and cure this damage. This model was recognised as limited not least because pain intensity and variance is not necessarily proportional to physical damage, and treatments for physical damage do not always relieve pain. Indeed many cases of chronic pain have no obvious cause. Recent research proffers instead a biopsychosocial model for understanding pain, recognising that it is multidimensional. While the role of physical processes is seen as important, the impact of psychological mechanisms (eg. beliefs, thoughts, feelings, behaviour) and social mechanisms (eg. disability, relationships, roles) are also acknowledged as influencing a person's experience of pain, and the impact it has on them. These facets have been found to be integrated on many levels, with changes in one dimension affecting others (Keefe and France, 1999). This biopsychosocial model offers two important implications. Firstly it acknowledges that because of this complex interplay of mechanisms no two people experience pain in the same way, and secondly it opens up more routes for treatment.

Sensing pain

The first stage of sensing pain involves the stimulation of nociceptors (receptors that sense pain). This stimulation leads to electrical impulses being sent to the spinal cord, via A or C fibres. A fibres are larger and conduct electrical impulses at high speed to inform of current tissue damage, while C fibres are smaller and conduct impulses slowly, acting as a message to prevent further tissue damage. These primary afferents synapse at the dorsal horn of the spinal cord. From here the pain message is passed to the brain through the spinal cord and the brainstem. These messages are 'interpreted' by the brain, being relayed to the thalamus and cerebral cortex, an area where higher thinking takes place. These messages also activate the hypothalamus, a part of the brain that processes emotions. This area is also responsible for releasing stress hormones in the body and limbic system, accounting for the emotional responses we have to pain, such as anxiety and distress. While the reflex arc at the spinal cord allows a fast reflexive behavioural response to pain, higher level 'thinking and emotional' processes are involved in initiating more complex responses, such as resting or avoiding further pain.

The 'gate control theory of pain' (Melzack and Wall, 1965) details how information sent to the brain from nociceptors and touch receptors interact at the dorsal horn. This interaction can act as a 'switch', whereby stimulation of touch receptors can moderate nociceptive impulses, almost overriding them. This accounts for why tactile interventions such as massage can help lower pain intensity. At the same time as receiving afferent pain information, the brain can also send out descending efferent messages to inhibit neurones at the dorsal horn from responding to nociceptor impulses. In this way the model proposes that interactions at the dorsal horn and brainstem can act as 'gates' moderating pain intensity. If these gates are 'open' then more nociceptive information is able to pass through, so the experience of pain is more intense. If the gates are 'closed' then the impulses are moderated and pain intensity is lessened.

Combined with the move towards a biopsychosocial view of pain, this theory offers an important assertion: that pain sensation is open to moderation, and how someone processes pain cognitively and emotionally can impact on how they experience pain physically. See *Chapter 1* for further details of the anatomy and physiology of pain.

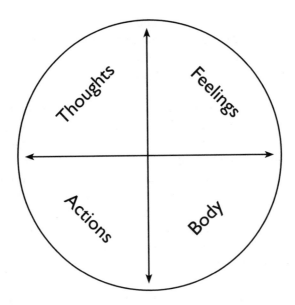

Figure 10.1: The hot cross bun analogy can be used to understand pain experiences and to explore areas for intervention.

Thoughts, feelings and physical sensations

Researchers have suggested a large overlap between physical pain processes and the thoughts, feelings, and actions we make in response (eg. van der Kolk, 1994; Chapman *et al*, 2001). It is not only physical processes that affect the way we experience pain but also the 'meaning' we give to it. In other words how we interpret the pain is influenced by our cognitive and emotional reaction to it. This is often guided by our past experiences and expectations.

The thoughts and feelings we have about things and the way we respond to pain are closely linked. How we experience pain is determined by how we make sense of it (thoughts), how it makes us feel (emotions), our physical bodily experiences, and the actions we take in response to the pain. This can be better understood through the 'hot cross bun' analogy. As *Figure 10.1* illustrates these four constructs are seen as being intrinsically connected (the cross), coming together to form someone's overall pain experience (the bun). This interaction means that difficulties or changes in one area can influence the others. This analogy is useful in helping to understand and explain a person's pain experience, and to explore interventions that may help to alter it.

Pain is often seen as something that is wholly physical needing a physical treatment to provide relief. Offering a psychological understanding or treatment may lead sufferers to infer from this that others do not believe their pain is real.

For this reason psychologically based understandings of pain and interventions need to be offered with clear explanation and reassurance.

As well as producing thoughts and feelings, pain can also produce a stress response, due to anxiety about the meaning and impact of the pain, as well as the intensity of the discomfort. While this demands emotional and cognitive reaction, it can also stimulate further physical sensations in the form of a 'fight or flight response'. This inbuilt response is activated when we feel threatened, and is the body's way of preparing itself to escape or face threat. This response is shown in a number of ways: physically, through muscle tension; cardiovascularly, through symptoms such as palpitations and a sense of 'panic'; gastrointestinally, through symptoms such as an upset or 'butterfly' stomach; cognitively, through preoccupation with thoughts of the threat or uncertainty about what actions to take; or emotionally, such as feeling frustrated or anxious. Chronic pain also causes stress through the impact it can have on areas of everyday life, for example on shopping, self-care, relationships or occupation. This all serves to create tension which opens the pain gates leading to increased pain intensity, causing further stress. This forms a vicious 'pain–stress' cycle (see *Figure 10.2*).

Coping strategies: The fear avoidance model

People's reaction to pain can be understood through looking at the interaction between their thoughts, feelings and physical experience of pain. Emotional and cognitive difficulties play a significant role in the level of distress and disability pain causes sufferers (Keefe *et al*, 1987), in their attempts to cope with the pain (Keefe *et al*, 1990) and their recovery (Julkunen *et al*, 1988; Waddell *et al*, 2002).

The fear avoidance model of chronic pain (Lethem *et al*, 1983) can be used to illustrate this link. The model proposes that people often assume that there is a direct link between damage and pain, interpreting hurt to be indicative of harm. In the chronic stage of pain, messages continue to be sent to the brain despite no ongoing tissue damage occurring, with the original cause having gone or remaining unclear. It is like a malfunction of the nervous system. Beliefs we have about pain (such as the idea that pain means harm) and the emotions it activates, both guide how we react to the pain and how we attempt to cope with it. The model depicts confrontation and avoidance to be the main responses to pain, with most people having a mixture of the two.

When first experiencing pain one may avoid certain activities (such as putting too much weight on a painful limb) to avoid further pain. As they recover most people push themselves to confront the pain by increasing the activity they have avoided. However, some people do not confront the pain but instead restrict their activities further and further. These people respond to pain with avoidance. This pain avoidance decreases exposure to pain, but it is a maladaptive (unhelpful)

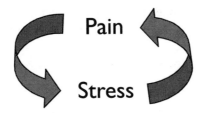

Figure 10.2: The pain–stress cycle.

response because it leads to further deconditioning, such as loss of muscle strength and flexibility, which serves to makes activity painful. Over time this avoidance fosters the expectation that activity will increase pain. This restriction of activities can lead to feelings of helplessness and depression, an association that is well supported within research (eg. Tate *et al,* 1994).

The explanation of why some people avoid rather than confront pain lies in how it is interpreted and responded to emotionally. Those who have a maladaptive response to their pain are likely to interpret pain as a threat. These people are then more likely to catastrophise about their pain (irrationally imagining the worst). This interpretation is likely to evoke feelings of fear, which in turn causes a stress response.

This interpretation and negative emotional response can elicit two behaviours; both are which are maladaptive strategies for dealing with pain. The first is akin to an anxiety response of focusing excessively on the pain, becoming vigilant in attending to pain symptoms (Bennett, 2002). This serves to increase pain and catastrophising. This response can be seen for example, in chronic pain patients who excessively seek health care support and evidence for their growing concerns, despite their situation remaining constant. The second response is avoidance of activities or interventions that risk inducing pain. This then leads to increasing levels of dysfunction and disability, as activities become increasingly painful due to their avoidance. This can build a sense of being at the mercy of pain, of feeling helpless and depressed. This response may be seen for example in patients who have poor engagement with services or interventions, seeming to appear unmotivated to change their situation. As health care professionals it is important to understand that responses to pain that can be troublesome may not be intentional, but are often born from cognitive and emotional distress.

The fear avoidance model demonstrates the importance of beliefs about pain and the feelings and behaviour these elicit. It also demonstrates why self-efficacy plays an important part in guiding how individuals experience, react to and recover from pain (Keefe *et al,* 1996, 1997).

To summarise, the following psychological factors have been identified as impacting on how pain is experienced, and can be pictured as acting to either close or open pain gates to increase or decrease the intensity of pain and the distress it can cause. Factors that decrease pain can be employed to form positive coping strategies.

Factors that increase pain include:

- attention to pain
- stress and tension
- negative thoughts or feelings, e.g. depression, anxiety, helplessness.

Factors that decrease pain include:

- distraction
- relaxation
- positive thoughts or feelings, eg. sense of control, achievement.

Cognitive-behavioural therapy (CBT)

Pain can cause even positive thinkers to have negative thoughts and to develop negative beliefs about their pain. This can increase pain intensity and decrease ability to cope. In time negative thinking patterns can affect other aspects of life, influencing, for example, relationships and mood.

Cognitive-behavioural therapy (CBT) involves identifying cognitions that are maladaptive (unhelpful) and challenging them. Because of the link between thoughts, feelings and behaviour, CBT can help alter each of these aspects to enable someone to hold a more positive view or interpretation of their difficulties, motivating them towards a more positive response to coping with their pain. This can help give a sense of control and lessen pain intensity.

There are four main steps to CBT. The first is to recognise and acknowledge the main thoughts and feelings an individual has about the pain and the behavioural response they make to it. The hot cross bun model is a useful aid for this, and can be completed by working through a specific example with someone, noting their thoughts, feelings and bodily sensations in the relevant area on the diagram. This can be done at difficult times or retrospectively. Patients can also record feelings in a diary to aid the identification of important patterns of thoughts and underlying beliefs. Questions that may act as helpful probes could include, 'What do you do when you are in difficulty?' 'What is the first thing that you think of?' 'Why is it important to you?' It is important that the individual recognises the link between how they think, what they feel and what they do.

Being aware of cultural differences can be helpful in enabling both therapist and client to build a common understanding of the client's experience of pain and the meaning it holds for them. This meaning can vary greatly and in non-Western cultures the experience of pain can be linked to religious beliefs and connotations. For example, pain could be seen as a punishment, as a test or trial, or as a symbol of survival and something to be rewarded (Pugh, 1991).

The second stage is to identify the key thoughts about pain that are maladaptive. Some people find it difficult to identify their thoughts, so it is sometimes easier to start by discussing any feelings that they experience as uncomfortable, or any behaviour that they recognise as unhelpful, and then examine what thoughts are behind these. Much research has been undertaken to identify key ways of thinking that can prove to be maladaptive. To illustrate, Burns (1980) identifies 10 common types of thinking that are often not helpful:

- All or nothing thinking: Seeing things in black and white. For example, if performance falls short of perfect, this is seen as a total failure.
- Overgeneralisation: Seeing a single negative event as evidence of a never-ending pattern.
- Mental filtering: Picking out a single negative detail and dwelling on it exclusively so that the vision of all reality becomes darkened.
- Disqualifying the positive: Rejecting positive experiences by insisting they 'do not count'. This can help maintain a negative belief.
- Jumping to conclusions: Making a negative interpretation even though there are no definite facts that convincingly support this conclusion. This includes assuming what others think.
- Magnification or minimisation: Exaggerating the importance of things, or inappropriately shrinking things until they appear tiny.
- Emotional reasoning: Assuming that one's negative emotions reflect the way things really are, adopting the view, 'I feel it, therefore it must be true'.
- 'Should' statements: Trying to motivate oneself with 'shoulds', 'shouldn'ts', 'musts' and 'oughts'. The emotional consequence for this can be guilt. When 'should' statements are seen as being initiated by someone else this can also create feelings such as anger, frustration, and resentment.
- Labelling and mislabelling: An extreme form of overgeneralisation. Instead of describing an error, a negative label is attached to the self such as, 'I'm a waste of space'. Alternatively when someone else's behaviour upsets you a negative label is attached to them.
- Personalisation: Erroneously seeing oneself as the cause of some external event.

The third step is to start questioning these thoughts by looking for more positive, and usually more rational, alternative views. For example, encouraging the individual to see their difficulties and situation in percentages or shades of grey rather than black and white, encouraging them to looking for evidence to support their conclusions, examining why they feel they 'should' do things and encouraging them to hold more flexible 'rules' for themselves. The use of affirmations can be useful in gaining acceptance of alternative views. These might include things like 'physical disability does not mean I am less valuable', 'circumstances are what they are but I can choose my attitude towards them', or 'I am learning to be honest with others, even when I am not feeling pleasant or nice'. Frequently repeating these affirmations can influence thoughts, feelings and behaviour.

The effectiveness of CBT is well researched with some good long-term results (eg. see Linton and Andersson, 2000). CBT is offered formally in a variety of settings on a one-to-one or group basis. The principles of identifying negative thoughts and looking for positive alternatives is something that can be employed both by people with chronic pain and by those around them.

Relaxation

Pain is stressful causing tension and distress, which in turn can increase pain. Relaxation can break this cycle, helping to build a sense of control over the pain. It can also relieve muscle spasms. Relaxation requires practice and there are many different tapes and exercises available, and different techniques suit different people.

Some people find it difficult to relax, have difficulty 'switching off' or find that they focus more on their pain. Practising initially when the pain is less, getting into a comfortable supported position, or using other strategies to lower pain levels beforehand may help. Relaxation techniques can also be used in conjunction with other interventions, for example using deep breathing with distraction techniques can be particularly effective. The following are some of the main techniques.

Deep breathing

One of the symptoms of the 'stress response' that can accompany pain is faster, shallower breathing. Deep breathing can help this and can be used separately, or as the basis for other relaxation techniques. It involves making full use of the diaphragm by breathing in through the nose, concentrating on the lungs slowly filling with air from the bottom, middle and then top until the top part of the body is tense, and then breathing out fully.

Progressive muscle relaxation

Progressive muscle relaxation involves working through the muscles of the body in sequence, gently tensing and relaxing them to focus on the difference between tension and relaxation. Any painful areas can be avoided.

Imagery

Imagery can be used to distract from the pain and to bring about a sense of 'escaping' to somewhere relaxing. This can be somewhere real or imaginary, such as a favourite place to visit or a picturesque scene built with the imagination. The scene can be built up through focusing on what may be there to see, smell, hear or touch.

Autogenic relaxation

Autogenic relaxation involves working through the muscles of the body to concentrate and visualise that they are increasingly heavy, warm and relaxed. This is particularly effective since heat often helps to ease pain.

STOP
Think of a patient in your clinical area who may have been feeling very anxious about ongoing pain. Do you think he or she may have benefited from some simple relaxation techniques?

Attention and distraction

Focusing on the physical sensations of pain can make it more intense. This attention gives the message to the nervous system that the pain sensations are important, thus opening the pain gates to allow more pain 'messages' through to the brain. This can lead to ruminating over the pain, as the cortex is receiving more and more pain impulses and these are increasingly experienced as distressing due to activation of the emotional and 'stress' response systems. This preoccupation also makes it is harder to cope constructively with the pain, because attention is focused on the pain itself rather than using learnt strategies.

Activities that take attention away from the pain can therefore be really beneficial, especially when the pain seems intense. An important role is in helping those in pain to divert attention away from the pain. Diversion techniques can include anything pleasant or requiring concentration from counting ceiling tiles or things in the room that are green, to puzzle books. The 'ABC' technique is a useful intervention, and involves picking a subject, anything from types of food to girls' or boys' names, then naming examples of the subject alphabetically. The subject should be something pleasant, and 'cheating' by using ideas that are only loosely associated with the subject is allowed, to ensure that the process is distracting but not distressing in itself.

Goal setting

Goals are a key to change. Having goals helps to motivate us and often helps us feel that we are living and not just existing. Working towards goals can give a sense of achievement, helping to increase self-efficacy and a sense of control over one's life. The process of setting goals is particularly valuable for people with chronic pain, and is often drawn upon by different health care professions. Chronic pain may cause people to feel unsatisfied with what they can achieve or manage in everyday life. They may have become focused on just 'coping', instead of being able to see a way forward.

For people with chronic pain having goals means determining what they do every day by planning in advance, rather than basing activity on how they feel or their level of pain. Goal setting allows people to be in control of their activities, planning what to do and how much to do at one time. Goal setting can also be a way of problem solving, allowing apparently big difficulties to be tackled by developing a step-by-step plan of how to move slowly towards a target or solution. There are many reasons why people may find it hard to set goals, and many will lie in the way people see their pain situation. However, setting and achieving goals, however small, seeks to increase self-efficacy through a sense of achievement. This can generate positive thoughts and feelings, which will decrease the pain experience. Goal setting involves four steps.

Step one

Step one is to identify an overall goal, eg. 'I want to improve my social life'. This can be simple or general. It can help to examine short- and long-term aims, in the areas of independence, relationships with others, household activities, relaxation, work, physical ability, leisure activity, or medication use.

Step two

The next stage is to break this overall goal into specific goals. For example, 'I want to see my existing friends more'. For people with chronic pain, having goals means determining what they do every day. Restate these goals to make them specific, measurable, achievable, realistic, have a time limit, and make them exciting and rewarding to provide motivation. In the example of seeing existing friends more, this could be restated as, 'I want to meet up with my friends at least twice a week beginning on Monday'.

Step three

The final stage is to break down specific goals into mini-goals, which are steps towards achieving a specific goal. Mini-goals in this example could include, 'Make a list of the people I know', 'Make a list of some places I can go', 'Phone a friend and arrange to meet next week'. It is important to think over and plan for any difficulties that may be encountered, and for these goals to be continually broken down until they are manageable. Failure can result in the opposite effect of eliciting negative emotions and thoughts, serving to decrease self-efficacy. These mini-goals should be achievable even on a day when the pain is intense, for it is on these days that having an 'action plan' to focus on is particularly helpful. It is equally important to include rewards each time a mini-goal is achieved to improve motivation and a sense of control over the pain. Rewards can be simple, such as doing something enjoyable, for example, listening to a favourite music track.

Goal setting can be thought of as a ladder with an overall goal at the top, and each rung being a mini-goal helping to get there. Each time a mini-goal is achieved it should help increase motivation and a sense of self-efficacy and achievement. It is important that difficulties are not seen as failures; other mini-goals or 'rungs' can be added as needed, and not achieving a mini-goal does not mean that all is lost. The setback will only be as far as one or two rungs of the ladder rather than being back at the beginning.

One goal that is particularly important to tackle is how to deal with a pain flare up or a 'bad pain day' effectively. While bad pain days may be helped by having achievable mini-goals to focus on, this situation could be problem solved directly by generating a 'flare up plan'. This could involve the same goal setting process with mini-goals that draw on interventions to help with the increased pain such as distraction, relaxation and reciting affirmations.

Interaction and communication

How others react to someone in chronic pain is an important factor in guiding how individuals understand and respond to their pain. Any thoughts about or responses to pain that are met with positive consequences or reinforcement by others are likely to increase. Similarly those met with negative consequences or feedback are more likely to decrease (Fordyce, 1976).

Therefore, it is important for those who interact with people who have chronic pain to be aware of how their responses can be interpreted and used to support or disqualify how individuals understand and respond to their pain. While it is important to recognise that someone is in pain, it is also important not encourage or reinforce pain responses or beliefs that are maladaptive. For example, responding to someone showing pain by doing things for them may encourage them to foster unhelpful interpretations of their pain, such as believing that their pain is damaging and they need help from others to avoid pain. This may in turn encourage them to ruminate about the pain, avoid certain actions, or feel helpless. Similarly, reinforcement and encouragement of a positive interpretation and response to pain can help people with chronic pain to cope more adaptively. For example, offering praise and encouragement for using positive coping techniques or for achievements made despite experiencing pain may mean that these coping strategies are repeated in the future.

Chronic pain affects not only pain sufferers, but also those around them. Experiencing chronic pain and the changes it may bring can put relationships with others such as family, friends, employers or health professionals under strain. Pain may lead people to become withdrawn or irritable, as well as affecting daily activities, goals and the roles they play in their relationships. However, many people with chronic pain also find that working with those close to them and including them in their experience of pain can bring a relationship closer together rather than further apart. Communicating with others is an important part of managing chronic pain effectively. Maladaptive patterns of communication, especially between patients and their close family, have been shown to affect levels of distress and pain intensity, as well as outcomes of treatment (eg. Tota-Faucette *et al*, 1993). People often find it difficult to communicate their needs, thoughts and feelings to others. Interventions such as communication and assertiveness training can help with this. Indeed the role of others in the development and perpetuation of chronic pain conditions, along with the effectiveness of communication skills training and relationship therapy, has drawn considerable empirical attention in recent years (eg. Kerns and Otis, 2003).

Interventions summary

- Explain the pain gate theory and the role of thoughts, feelings and behaviour. Emphasise that this means there are lots of things you can do to help control pain.
- Use CBT and challenge any maladaptive beliefs and behaviours sensitively.
- Teach relaxation and deep breathing.
- Teach distraction techniques.
- Be aware of the role of positive and negative reinforcement in interactions with others.
- Undertake communication training.
- When goal setting, devise achievable mini-goals.
- Help to establish a flare up plan.

Barriers to change

Many people have acute pain but not all end up with chronic pain, and some people with chronic pain seem to cope better than others. Chronic pain symptoms are largely seen as the product of many factors combining genetic, psychological and environmental vulnerabilities, as encapsulated by the biopsychosocial model of pain.

Some of these psychological vulnerabilities include depression, distress, or trauma that may have been in evidence prior to the onset of pain. While these may contribute towards developing chronic pain, they can also be a barrier to change. Because of the ability for maladaptive beliefs about one area of a person's life to evolve and 'spread' to being used to understand other areas of life, these factors can make targeting people's understanding of their pain and their ability to cope very difficult and sometimes futile. People often need time and space to deal with these underlying issues separately by being referred to other psychological services for help.

Conclusion

This chapter has concentrated on providing a brief overview of some of the practical interventions that can help manage chronic pain. It is however, important to acknowledge that chronic pain and the changes it may bring can have a deep and profound effect on a person's life. These changes can pose deeper psychological issues in many areas, including loss, identity and adjustment. Some individuals may need space to talk over these issues with help from psychological services, to assist them in making sense of what their pain experience means for them, and to help them move towards managing this. This help can be accessed both on its own or alongside other pain management interventions.

STOP

Does your area have a multidisciplinary pain management team? Do you know how to access it?

You may find spending some time talking to the clinical psychology team beneficial in helping you to understand the holistic picture of the patient in pain.

Implications for nursing practice

- As health care professionals it is important to understand that responses to pain may cause patients to seem unmotivated to change and this can be born out of fear and emotional distress.
- Nurses need to help reassure patients that for chronic pain hurt does not necessarily mean harm.
- Being aware of cultural differences can be helpful in enabling the nurse to build a common understanding of the patient's pain experience and the meaning it holds.
- Helping patients to set goals will help them gain a sense of control over their pain.
- Responding to pain by helping patients carry out the tasks of daily living may be unhelpful. It could encourage patients to believe that their pain is damaging to them.
- Reinforcing positive beliefs about pain and coping ability and being aware of not to reinforce maladaptive beliefs can help patients see that they can cope with life despite pain.
- Teaching basic relaxation techniques can help break the pain–stress cycle.

Key points

- The sensation of pain has a physical and emotional component.
- Thoughts and feelings and how we respond to pain are closely linked.
- Beliefs we have about pain and the emotions it activates both guide how we react to pain and how we attempt to cope with it.
- Chronic pain may cause people to feel unsatisfied with what they can achieve or manage in everyday life.
- Cognitive and behavioural techniques have an important role to play in the multidisciplinary treatment of pain.

References

Bennett R (2002) *Understanding Chronic Pain and Fibromyalgia: A Review of Recent Discoveries.* The Oregon Fibromyalgia Foundation. Available from: http// www.myalgia.com/chrpain.htm [Accessed: June 2006].

Burns MD (1980) *Feeling Good: The New Mood Therapy.* Avon Books: New York.

Chapman CR, Nakamura Y, Donaldson GW, Jacobson RC, Bradshaw DH, Flores L, Chapman CN (2001) Sensory and affective dimensions of phasic pain are indistinguishable in the self-report and psychophysiology of normal laboratory subjects. *J Pain* 2: 279–94.

Fordyce WE (1976) *Behavioural Methods for Chronic Pain and Ilness.* CV Mosby: St Louis.

Julkunen J, Hurri H, Kankainen J (1988) Psychological factors in the treatment of chronic low back pain. Follow-up study of a back school intervention. *Psychoth Psychosom* 50(4): 173–81.

Keefe FJ, France CR (1999) Pain: Biopsychosocial mechanisms and management. *Curr Dir Psychol Sci* 8(5):137–41.

Keefe FJ, Caldwell DS, Queen KT, Gil KM, Martinez S, Crisson JE, Ogden W, Nunley J (1987) Pain coping strategies in osteoarthritis patients. *J Consult Clin Psychol* 55: 208–12.

Keefe FJ, Caldwell DS, Williams DA, Gil KM, Mitchell D, Roberston C, Martines S, Nunley J, Beckham JC, Crisson JE, Helms M (1990) Pain coping skills training in the management of osteoarthritic knee pain: A comparative study. *Behav Ther* 21: 49–62.

Keefe FJ, Caldwell DS, Baucom D, Salley A, Robinson E, Tommons K, Beaupre P, Weisberg J, Helms M (1996) Spouse-assisted coping skills training in the management of osteoarthritis knee pain. *Arthritis Care Res* 9: 279–91.

Keefe FJ, Lefebvre JC, Maxiner W, Salley AN, Caldwell DS (1997) Self-efficacy for arthritis pain: Relationship to perception of thermal laboratory pain stimuli. *Arthritis Care Res* 10: 177–84.

Kerns RD, Otis J (2003) Family therapy for persons experiencing pain: Evidence for its effectiveness. *Seminars in Pain Med* 1: 79–89

Lethem J, Slade PD, Troup JD, Bentley G (1983) Outline of a fear-avoidance model of exaggerated pain perception-1. *Behav Res Ther* 21(4): 401–8.

Linton SJ, Andersson T (2000) Can chronic disability be prevented? A randomised trial of a cognitive-behaviour intervention and two forms of information for patients with spinal pain. *Spine* 25(21): 2825–31.

Melzack R, Wall PD (1965) Pain mechanisms: A new theory. *Science* 150: 971–9.

Pugh J (1991) The semantics of pain in Indian culture and medicine. *Culture, Med Psychiatry* 15: 19–43.

Tate D, Forchheimer M, Maynard F, Dijkers M (1994) Predicting depression and psychological distress in persons with spinal cord injury based on indicators of handicap. *Amer J Phys Med Rehabil* 73(3): 175–83.

Tota-Faucette ME, Gil KM, Williams DA, Keefe FJ, Goli V (1993) Predictors of response to pain management treatment: The role of family environment and changes in cognitive processes. *Clin J Pain* **9**(2): 115–23.

van der Kolk B (1994) The body keeps the score: Memory and the evolving psychobiology of posttraumatic stress. *Harvard Rev Psychiatry* **1**: 253–65.

Waddell G, Somerville D, Henderson I, Newton M (2002) Objective clinical evaluation of physical impairment in chronic low back pain. *Spine* **17**: 617–28.

Further reading and resources

Gatchel RJ, Turk C (1999) *Psychological Approaches to Pain Management: A Practitioner's Handbook*. Guilford Press: New York. This book provides a more detailed practical guide to psychological interventions for managing pain.

Linton SJ (2005) *Understanding Pain for Better Clinical Practice: A Psychological Perspective*. Elsevier: Edinburgh. This book gives an easy-to-read understanding of how pain is experienced and its implications for clinical practice.

Wells C, Nown G (1996) *The Pain Relief Handbook: Self-help Methods for Managing Pain*. Vermillion: London. This self-help book is aimed at patients and is recommended by the Pain Society.

www.psychnet-uk.com. This site has an excellent selection of explanations and resources accessible through the search engine facility.

CHAPTER 11

Complementary therapies and pain management

Avril Holland

This chapter explores complementary and alternative medicines (CAMs) in the context of health care, and specifically some of the various techniques that may be useful in managing both acute and chronic pain.

Pain management is an example of where the biomedical model can fall short. Patients in their need to alleviate pain become disillusioned with a lack of diagnosis and treatment and so seek alternative and complementary therapies in order to get some relief.

Many CAMs are provided by health care workers within the National Health Service (NHS) and an increasing number of general practitioners are offering CAMs as part of a treatment plan, especially in areas such as palliative care, pain clinics and neurology.

STOP

Thinking of your clinical area do any of your patients use complementary therapies? Is this assessed on admission?

What are your current beliefs about CAMs and how may these affect their use?

Chambers Concise Medical Dictionary (2000) defines complementary and alternative medicine together as 'The various systems of healing, including [those] not regarded as part of orthodox treatment..., especially when offered by unregistered practitioners...'.

STOP

Would you consider the above to be a reasonable working definition and if not give reasons for your decision.

You may have suggested that the terms 'alternative' and 'complementary' are interchangeable and that therapies are able to replace orthodox medical care.

More accurate definitions can be found in *Chambers Etymological Dictionary* (1963):

- Alternative: Offering a choice of two things. From the Latin 'alter' 'the other'.
- Complementary: Together making up a whole. From the Latin 'complere' 'to fill'.
- Medicine: Any substance used (especially internally) for the treatment or prevention of disease: The science or art of preventing, alleviating, or curing disease, ... as opposed to surgery or obstetrics. From either the old French 'medecine' or the Latin 'medicina', 'a medicine' or 'cure'.

STOP
Are you aware of any treatments that are sometimes used as an alternatives to medical treatments.

You may suggest that all non-conventional treatments are complementary, but that only a very small number can be considered in any way alternative to medical treatments and sought by patients as a first line therapy. Alternative treatments include acupuncture, osteopathy and chiropractic.

There is evidence of the use of 'complementary' treatments as the main source of disease management over thousands of years. See *Table 11.1* for an overview and time-line.

Philosophy of CAMs

Complementary practitioners work holistically, considering the totality of patients (body, mind and spirit), their lifestyle and demeanour, as well as their symptoms. Treatment aims to bring about homoeostasis (balance and harmony) and thus restore health.

According to the World Health Organization (1948) health is 'a state of complete physical, mental and social well-being and not merely the absence of disease or infirmity'. Holistic means 'emphasising the importance of the whole and the interdependence of its parts' (Readers Digest, 1984), which means considering the physical, mental, and emotional aspects of a person.

According to a House of Lords' Report (2000) 'Most CAM therapies also apply a non-Cartesian view of health, making less distinction between the body, mind and spirit as distinct sources of disease. The language used in CAM often tends to imply that all these dimensions of the human condition should be viewed in the same therapeutic frame. This often results in patients receiving a combination of treatments tailored to their specific needs. This is different from the medical approach which may involve prescribing a standard drug and a similar treatment regime for patients with the same underlying pathology.'

Dr Edward Bach (1886–1936), stated that 'health and happiness result from

Table 11.1: Brief 'time-line' of the development of complementary therapies

Date	Therapy
5,000 BC	Acupuncture in use
2,800 BC	Oils used in embalming – including cedar, frankincense and myrrh
2500 BC	Evidence of foot and hand massage treatments in Egypt
1240 BC	Moses used aromatic oils (e.g. olive, cinnamon)
1550 BC	Records describe the use of 700 plant medicines
0000	Frankincense and myrrh were gifts at the birth of Jesus
1st century	'De Materia Medica' by Dioscorides on herbal medicine – used until the middle ages
1st to 16th centuries	Due to the growth of science, folk medicine use declined in Europe
1653	Nicholas Culpepper wrote *The English Physician*
1770s	Anton Mesmer devised mesmerism – the foundation of hypnotherapy
1800s	Homoeopathy re-discovered by Dr Samuel Hahnemann
1804	Society of Trained Masseurs founded – later the Chartered Society of Physiotherapists
1820s	Dr Constantine Hering developed the Laws of Cure
1844	Faculty of Homoeopaths founded
1864	National Institute of Medical Herbalists founded
1892	Dr Andrew Taylor Still founded the American School of Osteopathy
1895	Daniel D Palmer devised chiropractic in Canada
1913	Dr William Fitzgerald (ENT surgeon) was experimenting with pressure on parts of the body to create an anaesthetic effect elsewhere
1917	Dr John Martin Littlejohn founded the British School of Osteopathy
1920s	French chemist, Gattefosse, developed modern aromatherapy
1930s	Dr Edward Bach, Harley Street physician, developed 38 plant-based remedies to balance state of mind,

being in harmony with our own nature, and doing the work for which we are individually suited', and that 'disease is the reaction to interferences' (fear, uncertainty, loneliness, despondency, over-care for others, over-sensitivity to influences and insufficient interest in present circumstances) (Howard, 1995). He also stated that 'disease is in itself beneficent' and that 'the very part of the body affected is no accident' (Bach, 1931). Taken together Bach seems to suggest that the way we react to circumstances is what causes disease, and by acknowledging the interference we can change our behaviour and get well.

Bach, Hippocrates and other statesmen of medicine suggest that our diet is related to health, and Hippocrates (460–377 BC) states that 'Our food should be our medicine. Our medicine should be our food'.

Dr Constantine Hering (1800–1880) determined three 'Laws of Cure', which state that healing progresses from within to without, from head to toe, from major organs to minor, and that symptoms clear in reverse order to their appearance. For example, a person with psoriasis and diverticulitis may notice that the digestive symptoms clear first, followed by the skin condition, with the legs and feet being the last part to clear.

It could also be argued that it has taken each person their lifetime to reach their current state of health, and some suggest that it takes as many months to get better as it took years to become ill.

Therapists generally work towards treating the causes of disease and restoring health, whereas orthodox practices tend to treat the manifestation of disease by treating the current symptoms.

Benefits and side-effects

Most CAMs are thought to work with the body to reverse a disease process and restore health by stimulating the body's own innate healing ability. Some therapies, such as hypnotherapy, alter the thoughts or patterns of behaviour that allow people to become or remain unwell. The healing process may cause a temporary exacerbation of the presenting symptoms, or a recurrence of old ones. Some patients feel energised, others relaxed and tired after a session, particularly after the massage therapies. Pain relief depends on the therapy but is often related to:

- The feeling of relaxation, which can reduce muscle spasm and release endorphins.
- An increased feeling of well-being and a perceived reduction in pain.
- Realignment and stretching of joints.

House of Lords Select Committee Report (2000)

Over the past two decades there has been a dramatic increase in demand for complementary treatments of all kinds, following media publicity and anecdotal evidence of benefit. This has led to a corresponding increase in the numbers of both therapies and practitioners, leading to concern and confusion over standards of training, practice, knowledge base and evidence of effectivity.

A report on CAMs was commissioned by the House of Lords in the 1990s, to investigate and report on all aspects of CAM, partly because of growing concern for the safety of the public (expressed by the medical establishment, professional organisations, individual therapists and the media) and partly due to information from the Prince of Wales' Foundation for Integrated Health (PoWFIH).

The House of Lords report, which was published in 2000, classified therapies into three groups, described their philosophies and claims, and made many recommendations designed to promote the safe practice of CAMs, while protecting both practitioner and customer.

The groupings and some of the major recommendations are given below.

Groupings of therapies

Group 1: Professionally organised therapies:

- osteopathy
- chiropractic
- acupuncture
- herbal medicine
- homoeopathy.

These therapies are based on individual diagnostic approaches.

Group 2 includes the popular therapies, that do not claim to diagnose ailments:

- aromatherapy
- Alexander technique
- flower essences
- healing
- Maharishi
- Ayurvedic medicine
- massage
- nutritional medicine
- reflexology
- shiatsu
- yoga
- hypnotherapy, meditation and stress therapy.

Group 3 includes those that seem to have little scientific foundation, but which aim to provide diagnostic information as well as treatment. There are two sub-groups:

Group 3a:

- Ayurvedic
- Tibb and traditional Chinese medicine
- cranio-sacral therapy.

Group 3b:

- crystal therapy
- iridology
- radionics
- dowsing
- kinesiology.

Thus groups 1 and 3a therapies are those that could be considered as alternative, and where practitioners are taught diagnostic techniques, and may be able to take clinical charge of a patient. Therapies in groups 2 and 3b identify, by various means, which systems, organs or glands are not functioning as well as they might or areas of the body that have been damaged in the past, and aim in most cases to stimulate the body's own internal healing mechanisms.

Recommendations from the report

The recommendations relevant to health care practitioners include:

- It should be ensured that there is evidence to substantiate any claims made for a therapy.
- Where there is evidence of therapeutic benefits of a therapy, then the public should have access to it, via medical practitioners and the NHS.
- Each discipline should have one professional body, bringing together all the current professional associations, with a clear structure, training standards, ethics, and continuing practitioner development opportunities/requirements.
- All undergraduates on medical courses should be exposed to a level of CAM, including how, when and why they may be used, and any potential dangers, sufficient to be aware of the choices their patients may make and to be able to 'deal with' those who may already be using CAMs.
- Royal colleges and other training establishments should support continuing professional development opportunities to ensure that students are able to become familiar with CAM.

- The Royal College of Nursing and the UKCC (now the Nursing and Midwifery Council) should work together and ensure that, when qualified, nurses are aware of the choices patients may make. Further, that as these bodies do not provide CAM training, they should compile a list of acceptable courses, so that nurses may obtain appropriate training.
- CAM practitioners should be familiar with other CAM disciplines.
- CAM practitioners should receive guidance on when to refer for medical care.
- More funding should be made available for suitable research to answer the questions: does it work, is it safe, is it cost-effective?
- NHS provision of CAM should be by referral from health care professionals to only those therapies that are well-regulated, whether in primary, secondary or tertiary care.
- The NHS should be the main information provider, including NHS Direct and Online.

Currently the majority of individuals using complementary care/therapy do so of their own accord and at their own expense. Many private health insurance schemes recognise reputable qualifications and will reimburse the cost of treatments (group 1 and some in group 2); some require medical referral and others do not.

STOP

Do your patients ask for advice on CAMs?
How would you advise a patient to access (safe, appropriate) therapy?

Why and how people use CAMs

It has been stated in the media that one in five of the population use, or have used, some form of complementary treatment. Some patients believe CAMs are more effective for their condition than conventional medical treatment.
  Other reasons given are:

- To take responsibility for their own health and healing.
- To stay well, reduce stress levels, recharge batteries.
- To support the body, alongside conventional medicine.
- As an alternative – a few people will turn their back on orthodox treatments altogether – and there have been some spectacular reports of recovery. See case study below.
- To avoid chemical drugs. CAMs are deemed more natural.
- To avoid polypharmacy and/or synthetic drugs and their side-effects.

- For symptomatic relief for common health problems, such as back pain, sciatica, migraine, strains and sprains, arthritis, tinnitus, irritable bowel syndrome, hay fever.
- To improve quality of life when the NHS only offers symptom control for chronic conditions such as osteoporosis, multiple sclerosis, chronic fatigue syndrome, head injury, and some cancer patients.
- To aid convalescence after illness, trauma and surgery.
- When there is 'something not right' but science is unable to identify the 'something'.
- For those born with disabilities such as cerebral palsy, Down's syndrome and spina bifida.

STOP

Think about when you might consider using CAMs. Can you think of someone who would benefit?

Case study

A lady walked into a consulting room with a slight limp. When asked the reason, she stated that 6 months previously she had been wheelchair-bound with multiple sclerosis, diagnosed with aggressive breast cancer and given 6 months to live. She continued, 'I decided to prove them wrong; I went to a retreat in Scotland, ate only fresh, organic foods and drank only spring water. I practised meditation and visualisation, enjoyed some fresh air and gentle exercise and here I am with no evidence of cancer [it had not shown on her latest mammogram] and feeling better than I have for years.'

Complementary therapies and nursing

Although only a small number of hospitals provide complementary therapies many nurses routinely incorporate them into their nursing practice. Massage, aromatherapy and reflexology in particular are increasingly being used. Nurses are pioneering the expansion of complementary therapies in the NHS.

In 1992 the UKCC (now the Nursing and Midwifery Council) recognised the growing use of complementary therapies within nursing practice and offered advice on the standards required of trained nurses using CAMS (Royal College of Nursing, 2003). The Royal College of Nursing Complementary Therapies Forum recognises the importance of education that includes:

- Course content that is appropriate for clinical practice.
- A period of supervision
- Formal examination that assesses knowledge and skills, ensuring that nurses are fit for purpose and able to obtain insurance.

Nurses are also reminded of the importance of working within the policy of their employing organisation and ensuring that any care they give is appropriate, effective and safe.

STOP

Does your clinical area have a complementary therapies policy/protocol?
Do you know how to access it?

Pain management

In theory, any (or all) of the therapies may help to reduce pain, because they help restore homoeostasis, so will affect pain where it is part of the disease process.

Therapeutic modalities

Complementary therapies generally fall into the following categories:

- Touch therapies, such as massage, aromatherapy and refloxology.
- Mind–body medicine, such as hypnotherapy, meditation and yoga.
- Manipulative and structural therapies, such as osteopathy, chiropractic and yoga.
- Postural techniques, such as the Alexander technique.
- Medicinal therapies, such as homoeopathy, herbal medicine and flower remedies.
- Oriental medicine, such as acupuncture and Chinese herbal medicine.
- Self-help, such as yoga, t'ai chi and meditation.

Some of the more common therapies are described here.

Acupuncture

Acupuncture is the most accepted of the therapies within medical practice, and there are recognised short courses for doctors, physiotherapists and nurses to enable its specific use for pain management.

Acupuncture originated in China and involves inserting small needles into various points on the body to stimulate nerve impulses. Traditional Chinese acupuncture is based on the idea of 'qi' (vital energy) which is said to travel around the body along 'meridians' which the acupuncture points affect. Western acupuncture uses the same needling technique but to affect nerve impulses and the central nervous system, to produce anaesthesia or analgesia.

Acupuncture is used in NHS pain clinics and physiotherapy departments and is found to be useful in the treatment of many chronic pain conditions and many acute problems related to muscle spasm.

Chiropractic and osteopathy

Chiropractic is used to treat musculoskeletal complaints through adjusting muscles, tendons and joints using manipulation and massage techniques.

Osteopathy is a system of diagnosis. Treatment may include soft tissue massage, rhythmical movements of joints, gentle releasing and stretching and high velocity thrust techniques.

To the patient there seems little difference between these two treatment modalities. Traditionally the main difference is that chiropractic theory suggests disease is due to an interrupted nerve supply and osteopathic theory suggests that disease is due to an impairment of the blood supply. Both treat similar problems, restoring and correcting bone/joint alignment, freeing any nerve compression (chiropractic), using soft tissue and deep massage techniques to restore alignment and improve circulation (osteopathy), and allowing the nerves to send the correct signals and/or blood to deliver the correct chemicals for the health of all tissues (and remove the waste products of metabolism). Tissues and structures that work properly do not send pain messages.

Many patients are referred to an osteopath or chiropractor by their general practitioner. Either therapy can be useful for:

- Headache.
- Painful arc syndrome (to release the joint and reduce shoulder pain).
- Low back or sciatic pain from trauma or misuse.
- Sporting injuries.
- Correcting pelvic misalignments, eg. following childbirth.

Homoeopathy, herbal medicine and aromatherapy

Homoeopathy, herbal medicine and aromatherapy use various parts of plants in different ways for medicinal purposes. The main differences are that herbal medicine uses only plant substances, homoeopathy uses plant, mineral and animal substances and aromatherapy uses the healing properties of essential plant oils.

Both herbal medicine and homoeopathic preparations are available as tablets, granules, powder, tinctures and creams.

Homoeopathy is a therapy based on the theory of treating like with like. Homoeopathic remedies use highly diluted substances that, if given in higher doses to a healthy person, would produce the symptoms that the dilutions are being given to treat. The cure of symptoms and eventually the disease is brought about by administering substances that produce symptoms similar to those that the person is experiencing. In assessing the patient homoeopaths often take into account a range of physical, emotional and lifestyle factors that contribute to the diagnosis. Homoeopathy reverses all the normal perceptions regarding substance, dosage and effectivity.

- The more dilute the remedy, the greater the effect (the law of infinitesimal dose).
- The remedy is chosen to treat the picture of symptoms (physical, mental and emotional) that manifest in patients, rather than a specific disease. (Illness is specific to the individual – and the model for holistic care.)
- The remedy of choice is the one that would produce the specific set of presenting symptoms if a well person took the original substance (the law of similars). For instance, cinchona bark (containing quinine) causes chills, fever and weakness – the symptoms of malaria – which it is used to treat.

Homoeopathic remedies are prepared by dissolving the substance (such as stinging nettle) usually in alcohol, to produce a 'mother tincture', then diluting further: 1:10 (X) or 1:100 (C) and shaking (succussing) them to produce a 1X or 1C potency remedy. The dilution process is sequentially repeated to produce further potencies – as far as 200C (1:100 x 200 serial dilutions) or even 1M.

A small range of homoeopathic tablets is available in many chemists and health food stores. Such remedies are usually 6C or 30C, in liquid form or as sublingual tablets. Arnica (Leopard's bane) is one of the commonest remedies, used to treat bruising and trauma. It may be taken before and after surgery to help the body recover from the effects of accidents or assaults (surgery is still traumatic to the body, even if it is planned). It may also be used to treat angina, and arthritic pain. Hypericum (St John's wort) may be used to treat nerve or shooting pains. Belladonna (deadly nightshade) is useful to treat throbbing or colicky pains, especially if there is fever present. *Urtica urens* (stinging nettle) is used to treat burning and stinging pains, eg. nettle rash, stings, shingles, gout, cystitis and burns.

There are four NHS homoeopathic hospitals in the UK, in London, Birmingham, Liverpool and Edinburgh.

Herbal medicine is a system of medicine that uses various remedies derived from plants and plant extracts to treat disorders and maintain good health. Herbalists are trained in the examination methods of conventional medicine but take a holistic approach to diagnosis and treatment, prescribing herbs and lifestyle changes and giving dietary advice.

Rather than treating a symptom in isolation herbal medicine seeks to restore what it calls 'the vital force' the body's own capacity to protect, regulate, renew and heal itself physically, mentally and emotionally. There are many hundreds of herbal preparations available to the public, prescribed in various ways such as capsules/tablets, infusions, ointments or tinctures, eg. comfrey (knit-bone) ointment is used to treat a wide variety of complaints, although not often specifically for pain relief. Hypericum (St John's wort) and lavender, as a tea, can be useful for nerve pain. Black cohosh can relieve muscle pains, including menstrual cramps. Ointments containing chilli pepper may be useful for relieving the pain of shingles. More complex or potent preparations are available only from qualified herbalists for individual patients. Remember that some modern drugs, such as aspirin and digoxin, were originally derived from plants (willow bark and foxglove, respectively).

STOP

We are all exposed to herbs on a daily basis. List the herbs that you use. The most obvious is peppermint used in toothpaste; many others are used in cooking.

Aromatherapy is a treatment that uses essential oils of plants in a controlled way to achieve balance and harmony in the human mind, body and spirit. The oils can be inhaled, used in massage, or occasionally ingested. They can be used to alleviate specific symptoms or as a relaxant.

There have been many studies of the properties of essential oils in the nursing press over recent years. Modern aromatherapy treatment generally combines the effects of the aroma from essential oils with the benefits of body massage to deliver them to the skin, where they are absorbed into the body. Many oils are available over the counter. They are thought to possess therapeutic qualities from the plant from which they have been extracted. Essential oils should always be diluted (in water, alcohol or vegetable oil or in lotions, ointments or creams) for use in baths, compresses or for massage. In the UK it is legal for doctors to prescribe oils on an ordinary prescription, however only medically qualified aromatherapists may prescribe oils to be taken internally. In the UK aromatherapists usually blend oils for individual clients/patients for clinic or home use.

Case study

A young boy with a fracture of his forearm had a compress of geranium, lavender and marjoram applied before attending hospital. This relieved the pain so successfully that the emergency department did not believe the arm was broken – until 10 minutes after the compress was removed.

Aromatherapy can be useful for pain associated with conditions as diverse as arthritis, burns (including those from radiotherapy), soft tissue injuries, trauma, colic and migraine. Oils with analgesic properties include:

* German chamomile
* eucalyptus
* lavender

- marjoram
- peppermint and spearmint.

Oils should be used with caution and under the guidance of a trained practitioner; while one drop of lavender (*Lavandula angustifolia*) on a pillow may aid rest and sleep, too much will result in wakefulness. Lavender is one of the very few oils that is generally safe to use neat on the skin. It can be used for pain relief for minor burns and scalds, cuts, spots, bites and stings. It is advisable to consult a good textbook when using oils at home as some oils are contra-indicated for certain health conditions such as hypertension and epilepsy as well as in pregnancy.

Massage

Massage is a systematic and scientific manipulation of body tissues performed with the hands for therapeutic effect on the nervous and muscular systems and on the systemic circulation.

Massage releases muscle tension, which relieves pain, as in 'rubbing it better'. There are various techniques, effleurage, hacking, cupping, etc., that can be used, depending on the disease and the intended outcome. Massage may be used alone or in combination with aromatic oils to enhance its relaxation and pain-relieving effects. Massage may be to a specific area of the body, such as the lower back for women in labour, or more generalised over the whole body. Massage should not be performed over any area of inflamed tissue.

Reflexology

Reflexology is a system of massage of the feet and, less commonly, the hands based on the idea that there are invisible zones running vertically through the body, so that each organ has a corresponding location in the foot. It has also been claimed to stimulate blood supply and relieve tension. According to Sullivan (1994), 'reflexology does not cure illness, or even diagnose, it simply stimulates the body's natural healing ability'.

The rationale is that the two feet together represent the head and torso of a person, with each part of the foot corresponding to (reflecting) a specific area of the body, e.g. the spine along the medial edges and limbs along the lateral edge of the feet. By massaging the feet an effect can be demonstrated in the body. There are many theories as to why reflexology works, such as touch (releasing oxytocin and/or endorphins), energy (working meridian points), increase in circulation (thereby delivering more oxygen and nutrients to the tissues), nerve stimulation, relaxation and release of stress, gravitational congestion (where toxins within the body fall to the lowest point – the feet) (Mackereth and Tiran, 2002). In order to relieve pain a therapist would work the reflex corresponding to the area where the pain is felt, plus the adrenal gland (to encourage natural steroid production), the pituitary gland and hypothalamus (to encourage the release of oxytocin) and the spine in an attempt to alter the pain message.

Reflexology is a popular therapy for nurses to learn and use.

Case study

A middle aged lady needed to attend a meeting following a dental extraction. After receiving a reflexology treatment of two minutes duration on the jaw and tooth and adrenal areas of her hand, she reported that she was pain free and that the effects lasted for three hours. The patient felt that the effects lasted as long as relief from 1g of paracetamol and without the side-effects.

Hypnotherapy

Hypnotherapy is an altered state of consciousness induced by deep relaxation. This state of relaxation is bought about by patients themselves and can only be induced by another person if the recipient requires it.

There is mounting evidence that the mind really can control matter and hypnotherapy can be effective for the relief of acute or chronic pain from any cause. Its benefits are mainly related to the release of muscle tension which is associated with all painful conditions. Self-hypnosis techniques can be taught to empower patients to manage their own pain and is used in many pain clinics as part of a pain management programme.

Shiatsu

Shiatsu is a Japanese word meaning healing with hands, literally 'finger pressure'. It is based on the principles of acupressure, ie. chi (life energy) circulates around the body along 14 meridians (two central meridians, drawing chi through the torso and 12 mirrored pairs along the symmetric halves of the body). Shiatsu uses a combination of hand pressure and manipulative techniques to achieve diagnosis and treatment. The relevant meridian points are stimulated by pressure from fingers and thumbs, elbows, knees or feet, with the intention of calming overactive energy channels or activating sluggish or blocked channels and adjusting the body's physical structure.

Healing

Healing is a system of spiritual healing, sometimes based on prayer and religious beliefs. It attempts to tackle illness through non-physical means, usually by directing thoughts towards an individual. It often involves the laying on of hands. Reiki also involves the laying on of hands and to the patient both appear the same. The practitioner acts as a channel for universal energy and transmits it to the patient via the hands. This beneficial energy has the intention of restoring balance where there are imbalances, ease where there is disease and reactivating a patient's own healing ability.

Some therapists rest their hands on the patient, others work solely about one to two inches from the body, within the aura (or energy field that surrounds every living thing). Treatments can take place anywhere, anytime and there are no cautions or contra-indications. For the relief of pain therapists may focus on the area where the pain is felt and the nervous system and help the patient relax.

Reiki is a Japanese technique for stress reduction, relaxation and healing. It is based on the idea that an unseen life force energy flows through us and is what causes us to be alive. The practitioner acts as an energy channel for the recipient. The energy is drawn by a need or imbalance within the patient. The channelled energy enables the body to speed up its own healing process. Reiki is thought to work at all levels, physical, mental, emotional and spiritual. As well chronic injuries it can treat problems such as asthma, eczema and headaches.

Conclusion

Some complementary therapies, eg. acupuncture, osteopathy and chiropractice have been used for the relief of pain for a number of years. Many of the CAMs mentioned in this chapter have a place in helping patients to take control and manage their pain more effectively and in some cases to reduce it. Nurses are key practitioners in actively integrating a variety of CAMs into their clinical practice. Adherence to strict local policies and guidelines and the availability of data from robust clinical studies will only help to implement and enhance this area of nursing and improve the service provided to the patient with pain.

Implications for nursing practice

- None of the remedies in this chapter is intended to replace medical diagnosis and treatment; anyone intending to support patients and clients wishing to use complementary therapies should always recommend consulting a qualified and insured practitioner.
- In order to practise a complementary therapy nurses need to have undergone some form of recognised training and have proof of having successfully completed a course.
- A stated amount of time has to be set aside for therapies during which other practices must take a lower priority.
- Nurses should not deny patients treatment because they do not believe it will work.

Key points

- One in five of the population have used complementary therapies. An increasing number of GPs are using complementary therapies as part of a treatment plan.
- Some patients believe therapies to be more effective than medical treatments.
- Pain management is an example of where the biomedical model can fall short.
- The House of Lords commissioned a report to investigate and report on all aspects of CAMs.
- Nurses should accept and encourage their use in selected patients.

References

Bach E (1931) *Health Thyself*. CW Daniels: Saffron Walden.

House of Lords Select Committee (2000) *6th Report on Complementary and Alternative Medicine (CAM)*. HMSO: London.

Howard J (1995) *The Work of Edward Bach. An Introduction and Guide to the 38 Flower Remedies*. Wigmore Publications: London.

Mackereth PA, Tiran D (Eds.) (2002) *Clinical Reflexology: A Guide for Health Professionals*. Churchill Livingstone: London.

Readers Digest (1984) *Readers Digest Great Illustrated Dictionary*. Readers Digest Association: London.

Royal College of Nursing (2003) *Complementary Therapies in Nursing, Midwifery and Health Visiting Practice*. London: Royal College of Nursing

Sullivan K (1994) *Alternative Remedies*. Harper Collins: London and Glasgow.

World Health Organization (1948) *WHO Constitution*. Available from www.who.int/about/en [Accessed 2 January 2007].

Bibliography

Dimond B (1998) *The Legal Aspects of Complementary Therapy Practice. A Guide for Health Care Professionals.* Churchill Livingstone: Edinburgh.

Ernst E (Ed.) (2001) *The Desktop Guide to Complementary and Alternative Medicine.* Harcourt Publishers: London.

Lawless J (1993) *The Encyclopaedia of Essential Oils.* Element: London.

Ody P (1995) *The Herb Society's Home Herbal.* Dorling Kindersley: London.

Shepherd D (1989) *Homoeopathy for the First Aider.* Daniel CW: London.

Westwood C (1992) *Aromatherapy: A Guide for Home Use.* Amberwood Publishing: Rochester, Kent.

Woodham A, Peters D (1997) *The Encyclopaedia of Complementary Medicine.* Dorling Kindersley: London.

Worwood VA (1991) *The Fragrant Pharmacy.* Bantam Books: London.

Useful websites

www.chiropractic-uk.co.uk
www.mctimoney-chiropractic.org
www.osteopathy.org.uk
www.homeopathy-soh.org
www.nimh.org.uk
www.ifparoma.org
www.reflexologyforum.org
www.aor.org
www.bsch.org.uk
www.nsph-hypnotherapy.co.uk/
www.shiatsusociety.org
www.gerneralshiatsucouncil.org
www.nfsh.org.uk
www.snu.org.uk
www.acupuncture.org.uk
www.reikiassociation.org.uk

Index

A

abdominal pain 26
Aβ fibres 3–4
acupuncture 71–72, 151–152
acute pain 37–50
  assessment of 25–36
  drug management of 38–42
  in elderly patients 47
  psychological management of 48
Aδ fibres 3–4
adjuvant analgesia 67, 85–86
adolescents
  pain in 105–106
aerobic exercise 118–119
alternative medicine
  see CAMs
anti-arrhythmics 20
anti-spasmodics 20
anticonvulsants 19
anxiety 130
aromatherapy 152–155
aspirin 16
assessment of pain 27–29
  factors affecting 27–28
  in palliative care 79–80
autogenic relaxation 135

B

behavioural training 69–70
biopsychosocial
  approach to physiotherapy 115
  model of pain 127
body charts 31–32
bone pain 81

C

CAMs 143–160
  and nursing 150–151
  benefits of 146
  philosophy of 144–146
  side-effects of 146
  time-line 145
cancer pain
  specialist analgesics 86
categorical scales 30
C fibres 3–4
chest pain 26
chiropractic 72, 152
chronic pain
  assessment of 51–62, 65–66
  psychological aspects of 127–142
  psychosocial problems 64
  types of 64–65
cognitive-behaviour therapy 120,
    132–134
complementary and alternative medicines
  see CAMs
coping strategies 130–132
corticosteroids 20
CRIES assessment tool 105
cyclo-oxygenase 16–17

D

deep breathing 134
descending modulation 5–6
distraction techiques 135–136
dorsal horn 4

E

endogenous opioid peptides 3–4
entonox 41
  contra-indications 41–42
epidural analgesia 44–47
  side-effects 46–47
ethical issues
  and cancer patients 91
exercise 114, 116–119

F

Faces Scale 30–31
fear avoidance 130–132
first-pass metabolism 13

G

gate control theory of pain 7, 128
goal setting 136–137
guided imagery 103–104

H

healing 156–157
herbal medicine 152–155
homoeopathy 152–155
hypnosis 71
hypnotherapy 71, 156

I

imagery 135
inhaled preparations 44

J

joint
  manipulation 113–114
  mobilisation 113–114

L

local anaesthetic
  for pain management 39–40
  side-effects of 40

M

manual therapy 111–114
massage 111–112, 155
McGill Pain Questionnaire 31, 80
meaning of pain 129–130
multidisciplinary team
  approach to chronic pain 65–66
muscle relaxation 135
musculoskeletal pain 65

N

neonates
  pain control in 104–105
nerve block 21, 68
neuropathic pain 2, 38, 53, 65, 80
neurotransmitters 3
NMC Code of Professional Conduct 60
nociceptive pain 2, 38, 53
nociceptors 128
non-malignant pain
  management of 63–76
non-opioid analgesics 16
  in palliative care 82
NSAIDs 16, 40, 101
  contra-indications 40
  side-effects of 41
numerical rating scales 30, 57

O

opiate analgesia 38–39
  side effects of 39
opioid
  analgesia 17–18
    and addiction 84
    and breakthrough pain 84
    in children 101–102
    in palliative care 82
    side-effects of 83–84
    spinal 21–22
    tolerance to 84
  rotation 84
oral analgesia 42
osteopathy 72, 152

P

pain
  anatomy of 1–9
  assessment
    in children 95–100
    tools 29–33, 56, 80
  at the end of life 90

descriptors 52
diaries 57
impact on family 89–90
management
  in children 95–110, 100–104
  of acute 37–50
misconceptions about 58–59
pharmacological treatment of 11–24
physiology of 1–9
quality of 57–58
questionnaires 80
receptors 2
relief
  non-pharmacological methods of
    102–104
sensation of 128
with no apparent cause 53
pain–stress cycle 130–131
palliative care 77–94
paracetamol 16, 41, 101
parenteral preparations 42–43
patient controlled analgesia 12, 43
pharmacokinetics 13–14
pharmacological treatment
  routes of delivery 11–12
physiotherapy 69, 111–124
picture scales 30
play therapy 104
prescribing principles 14–15
preventive approach
  to analgesia 67
protein binding 13–14
psychosocial problems
  and chronic pain 64

R

rectal preparations 42
reflexology 72, 155–156
Reiki 157
relaxation 70, 103, 134–135
response to injury 7

S

Shiatsu 156
soft tissue
  mobilisation 112–113
  pain 81
spinal
  cord 4
    stimulation 68
  opioids 21–22
spinorecticular tract 5
spinothalamic tract 5
strengthening exercises 117–118
stretching exercises 117
surgery
  for pain control 69

T

topical preparations 21, 44
total pain 87–89
transcutaneous electrical nerve stimula-
    tion (TENS) 68, 104
treatment modalities 42–47
tricyclic antidepressants 19

V

verbal rating scales 57
visceral pain 65, 80
visual
  analogue scales 30, 56–57
  displays of pain 32

W

WHO analgesic ladder 14–15, 66,
    81–82, 87

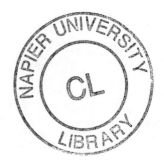